Francis Warner

The Study of Children and their School Training

Francis Warner

The Study of Children and their School Training

ISBN/EAN: 9783337215729

Printed in Europe, USA, Canada, Australia, Japan

Cover: Foto ©Paul-Georg Meister /pixelio.de

More available books at **www.hansebooks.com**

THE STUDY OF CHILDREN

AND THEIR SCHOOL TRAINING

THE

STUDY OF CHILDREN

AND THEIR SCHOOL TRAINING

BY

FRANCIS WARNER, M.D. (Lond.)

F.R.C.P., F.R.C.S. (Eng.)

Physician to and Lecturer at the London Hospital; Physician to
the Royal Albert Orphanage; formerly Physician to the
East London Hospital for Children
Honorary Member of the Hungarian Society of Public Health
at Budapest

New York

THE MACMILLAN COMPANY

LONDON: MACMILLAN & CO., Ltd.

1898

PREFACE

—◆◇◆—

THIS work is addressed chiefly to teachers, parents, and others in daily contact with children; but contains information that is likely to interest those engaged in directing education, philanthropy, and other forms of social work as well as those concerned with mental science.

The book has been written in the hope of aiding an advance in the care of children, and in the practice of educational methods, by promoting a more exact study and classification of the children to be cared for and trained; while giving an account of some conditions of childhood in its many varieties as seen from the standpoint of the observer who records what he sees as in other branches of physical science. For the purposes of observation, a clear account of the points to look at, what to look for, and what may be seen, normal or subnormal, forms the alphabet of our subject.

Child study has of late years been actively carried on in America and in other countries. The psychological researches of many American, and some English and German inquirers, are well known, and give most interesting records of the sayings and doings of young children, and their modes of thought and expression. In the psychological laboratory investigation has shown something of the laws of mental fatigue, and the reaction of the senses on the brain. The application of such knowledge, however, as well as the means of devising special methods in training needs, as a scientific basis, a fuller understanding of the groups of children to be educated, and the means of discriminating and describing them. Considerable differences are to be found among observers, both in the purpose of their studies, the points of view from which their work is undertaken, and the methods of procedure and description adopted.

Problems in child study may be looked at from different points of view; as mainly psychological, or as mainly physical questions, with the determination to follow the methods of observation, and the modes of description used in the conduct of biological study and the physical sciences; in the latter case it is important to describe phenomena by the use of terms indicating what we see and such as are employed in physical investigation. I think the best results will be obtained by keeping the two methods distinct, and suggest that in the scientific (physical) study of children in their modes of brain-action, and bodily conditions, we should describe what we see, and employ no terms implying results of consciousness and states of feeling. Child study conducted by any method is advantageous as directing attention to the individual child; it increases knowledge of child life, and tends to cultivate a fellow-feeling with the child as an object of interest.

I shall here use points for observation which I began to study twenty years ago, indicating brain-power and mental expression, such as render it possible to give descriptions of children, as of other living things, by describing facts seen. The study of such observations shows many new relations among growth, movement, and mental power. The principles used in biological study and natural history are here applied to child study.

In 1888 a committee was formed by the British Medical Association to study school children as to their mental and physical status, and in conjunction with medical men on that committee, and others, I was enabled to examine individually 100,000 children upon a fixed plan, taking a written description on a schedule for each child in any one point subnormal, or reported by the teacher as dull or backward.

Groups of boys and girls can be studied when their classification is arranged on a basis of points observed in individual children. Observation shows the child's strong points which should be cultivated, as well as his weak ones which must be combated. The interaction of classmates on one another may be observed by the teacher who observes the individual child under varied conditions. The importance of what have been called eye-mindedness and ear-mindedness, as well as action of the hand controlled through the eye, becomes emphasised to the mind of the observer.

Some generalisations, in the form of Propositions concerning Childhood, are given in the last chapter; it seems possible to attain a working consensus in interpreting much that we see for the practical purposes of education and the care of children. When the groups of children to be cared for are clearly discriminated, the educational methods needed for each can be more readily worked out.

Studies in psychology often emphasise the great mental differences among children; observation of the children themselves shows points of resemblance and difference, normal and subnormal, by which they may be grouped and compared.

F. W.

5 PRINCE OF WALES TERRACE,
KENSINGTON, W. LONDON.

NOTE OF EXPLANATION

In case the system of grading pupils by Standards in use in the London schools in which Dr. Warner made his examinations is not perfectly familiar to all his readers, it should be stated that bright children at six years of age should be found in Standard I.; at seven in Standard II.; at eight in Standard III.; at nine or ten in Standard IV. or V.; at eleven or twelve in Standard VI. or VII. Possibly the majority of children will be from three to six months behind this estimate.

CONTENTS

CHAPTER I

CHAPTER II

ix

CHAPTER III

PAGE

Description of the brain. Nerve-cells; nerve-fibres, nerve-force, and nerve-currents. Movement resulting from brain-action. Analogy to a galvanic cell. Nerve-fibres passing up to the brain, and others passing from it to the muscles. Diagram of brain, nerves, and muscles. Nerve-centres or parts of brain act separately. Every movement is due to action of a nerve-centre. A series of movements indicates a series of nerve-centres acting, controlled through the senses. Stimulation producing movement. All expression of the action of mind is by movement. Expression of emotions. A child in sleep. Brain-action requires food and stimulation through the senses. Brain-action observed in movements of infant. Spontaneous movements in new-born infant; also in young animals and seedling plants. Brain-centres act separately in infant. Movements when a month old: at three months, some control through the senses. Associated movements of the hands. At five months, movement regulated through eye and ear. At three years, signs of mental action and memory. A case. Infantile brain-action evolves as mental expression. Action in brain corresponding to regulated movements. The dawn of mental faculty. Case, action adapted by circumstances at three years. Kind of movement seen in the infant.

CHAPTER IV

Studying children: observing in place of questioning the child. Examples. Case: a well-made boy, exhausted. How to observe. Points to look for; development, nerve-signs, nutrition. Schedule for recording observations. Fix your ideas of the normal type. The head: parts for observation; common defects; measurements. Study good statuary. The face: types. Separate features. Nose. Palate. Ears. Growth.

Nerve-signs. General balance. Expression in the face, facial zones. Analysing a face. Eye-movements; muscles of the eye, the pupil. Head, postures and movements. Hand-balance as an index of the brain. The normal straight hand posture.

LIST OF ILLUSTRATIONS

LIST OF TABLES

LIST OF CASES

xviii

THE STUDY OF CHILDREN

AN educational system has been introduced, and made available for all classes, in order that young people may grow up with their faculties well developed, fitting them to become useful men and women in their future social life. But, while looking at the scope and the public usefulness of a system of education, we must remember that children differ greatly in health and strength and in mental faculty; education should therefore be adapted to the special needs of the individuals. Children of school age, *i.e.* from three to fourteen years, form about one-fourth part of the population. We shall see that there are many classes and varieties of children, whose needs must be studied; while the bodily strength and mental faculty of an individual will be shown to vary at different age-periods, and according to the environment. Hence, child study must be a matter of primary interest

B   I

to the teacher and others engaged in the care of
children, as affording a basis for the methods of education; giving a source of perpetual interest to work
in school, an interest in the individual child, and a
reasonable means of working out, in practice, the
best that can be done with the child in various
phases of life.   Without an intimate knowledge of
children the teacher may have difficulty in the presence of a peculiar pupil.

Case 1. A boy, eight years of age, in a prepara-
tory school, was said to be so dull at learning Latin,
that it was thought impossible to continue the attempt to teach him.   He was healthy and well made;
he showed no signs of mental defect, and was, otherwise, quick and bright.   He had learned to read well
and read story-books for pleasure.   I noticed that,
in reading, he followed the words on the printed line
by moving his head, not moving his eyes in their
orbits; this did well enough for story-reading, when
he skipped much of the page.   Moving the head, in
place of turning the eyes, did not admit of sufficient
accuracy for studying Latin.   Some attention to eye-
drill soon removed all the difficulty complained of,
and the boy made good progress.   This cause of
mental dulness will be referred to again; the case
serves to illustrate the usefulness to teachers of personal observation.

Children in a school class usually vary; each has

his own peculiarities. A rough classification may be made of the temperament, disposition, and mental characteristics of each, and still there remain individual peculiarities, which should be recognised as a guide to training. Some children are active in temperament, kindly in disposition, and quite up to average for their age in mental ability; an individual of that class may give trouble by outbursts of passion and periods of mental confusion; such pupils will need careful consideration and management.

Case 2. A girl was doing a sum, simplifying a compound fraction quietly and correctly, line by line: then the forehead puckered and the eyebrows were knit together, while the face flushed and the angles of the mouth became depressed; at the same time, the fingers of the right hand, which held the pen, twitched, and she wrote $114-16=24$. Writing quickly on a piece of paper $\frac{114}{16}$ and putting it before her was immediately followed by the face clearing, while the figure 98 was at once filled in; the work was continued without a word said; thus a storm was prevented by rapid observation of the signs accompanying mental confusion.

Observation and study of children as to their mental status will add power to the position of the teacher, to be exercised for the benefit of children. To observe and to think does not suffice to complete the

method of child study; we should be able to describe
in words what we see, both as an aid to accurate
thinking, and as a means of expressing the grounds
of an opinion, formed as to the status of the child
and the effects of training. Accuracy in thus forming an opinion may do much to save friction between
the school and the parent, and to establish a good
understanding.

Case 3. A boy was sent to Kindergarten; on returning home at midday, it was always difficult to make him
take his dinner; he talked much, turned away from his
food, was cross, nothing was pleasing to him; he was
restless and looked full under the eyes; at night he
talked in his sleep, in the morning he was tired and did
not want to get up. He was a healthy, well-made child.
In school he was reported as bright and eager, did as
he was told, liked the games, and did not seem tired.
The teacher saw him bright and happy, when occupied
and under the stimulus of school and companions; the
parents saw him after such stimulus was removed.
Each account of the child was true; they were taken
under different circumstances.

Case 4. A boy attending an elementary school was
brought to me by his mother, because he was troublesome, did not do his work, and was always in disgrace
and punishment, and she did not know what to do with
him. I observed at once that he had a cleft upper lip,
which had been closed by a surgeon, but the scar

remained. Knowing the frequency of several defects in the same child, and that the brain in such cases is often, but not always, badly made, I examined him with care. The boy had a defect of his heart, and his brain was ill-developed. Advice was given that he should continue at school, and that the teacher should be informed as to his condition, that he might be kindly treated, and not expected to pass examinations. This boy has a right to the benefits of education; they afford the best chance of his improvement, and of preventing him from becoming a failure in life. Such cases are common.

As to method of observation and study, I have to explain, as shortly and clearly as possible, how you can observe children for yourselves, and think about your observations with advantage. The observations you make for yourselves will always be of use to you; in making observations we can all agree; the inferences drawn therefrom may differ according to the aspects in which they are considered, and the special experience brought to bear. The points to be defined for observation are grounded upon my personal observation of 100,000 children who were seen individually. Some principles which underlie accurate observation and description will be explained, to help you in planning what you will do and what to look at.

A certain amount of training is necessary to make a good observer; the teacher who has to give object lessons or teach natural history needs not only to be an accurate observer himself, but also to be capable of training children to observe, *i.e.* to see and to think about what they see. Looking at a buttercup flower, you may name it and say where it grows; that it is of no particular use to the farmer, but is a very pretty flower; that it is a yellow flower and without scent. Then you will show the parts of the flower, the five parts that are coloured, showing that they are separate from one another, and all alike in size and in form. So you proceed to look at all the parts of the flower, their number, size, form, the proportions of the parts, and you compare them. Occasionally you will find a flower in which the coloured parts (petals) are not all of the same size, and with some variation of colour; points a little different from the usual and below the normal.

Now look at a kitten : it may be more difficult to demonstrate than the flower, because it is alive and full of movement; but more interesting, because it does move, and shows some instinct or intelligence. You proceed, as with the flower, to look at its body, each limb and its parts, the ears and the tail, the claws, etc. We look at each part of the kitten. Its movements are more interesting points : movement indicates its playfulness, the instinct, and something like intelligence in the cat : movements tell you more of the disposition and character of the cat than its colour, the length of its hair, and its ears and tail. In studying a living thing we observe its parts, and in a living animal we observe movements in its parts: we must study the child in the same way.[1] I shall call your attention to the body of the child, its height, weight, and proportions as a whole, and to the physiognomy or proportioning of the head and separate features and parts.

Over and above the observation of the body, as a still object, you must look at the movements of its parts, which are the direct outcome of action in the brain and nerve-system; thus you may study growth of body and action of brain, as you look at the child and think about his mental action and the interaction of the mind and body. In studying a child, to ascertain all you can about his mental disposition, you must look at him for the purpose of seeing all possible signs of his brain action, and how it is controlled and affected by circumstances: by studying individual pupils continuously you will acquire valuable experience and be able to form generalisations from your observations, as a basis of mental study. When you have learnt to recognise and describe the points, seen in the well-developed but nervous child, examples will remain in your memory, and in your note-book, and you will find that they are usually quick in mental action; affectionate, but sometimes passionate, gregarious in social habit, and give difficulty in school on account of their over-mobility,

[1] See "Anatomy of Movement: A Treatise on the Action of Nerve-Centres and Modes of Growth," by the author. The Macmillan Company.

excitability, fidgetiness, and liability to fatigue and headaches.   These facts will stimulate your interest in these
"troublesome children" and show the origin of some of
their faults.   I have seen such children in school sit
together at the back-desks of the classroom, where their
quick wits enabled them to complete their sums or exercise quickly; while their spontaneous mobility predisposed them to be the playful, talkative, laughing pupils
of the class.   I shall put before you the points, in
detail, which you may see and describe in the child.

Besides describing what you see in the child, I think
you will gain much by giving a general description in
your own words, indicating the mental action you may
observe in the pupil's words and work, and compare
this with points seen in the body and action of the child.

Case 5. I have seen a well-built, intelligent child,
who was interested in and quick at arithmetic, make an
absurd mistake.   The sum was to reduce six million
inches to miles, yards and feet: it was written thus :

$$12 \underline{|6,000,000} \text{ inches}$$
$$3 \underline{|500} \qquad \text{feet}$$
$$166''2 \qquad \text{yards} \qquad Ans. \text{ 166 yd. 2 ft.}$$

The purely mental work is correct; the first line
was drawn wrongly, the eye did not correctly guide
the hand.   It was, doubtless, extremely careless of the
child; but if you scold her, she will wriggle and flush
and look like crying; that does but little good.   Rather
look at the child as you work out a sum on the black-

board, note if the eyes are moved accurately and steadily towards the figures and lines of the sum; again, note if she move her hands and fingers accurately in imitation of yours when doing physical exercises. Want of control of the hand through the eyes may produce mistakes taken for mental faults.

Making an observation is, primarily, an act of seeing, and appreciating what you see; after observing you need to describe what you have seen. Seeing teaches much; describing what you see will add accuracy to your work and enable you to acquire a sound experience, which you can compare with that of others and correct from time to time. The points most commonly observed in the body and brain action of children are described in Chapters II., III., VI., while to aid the description of points below the normal a list of such signs is given and a schedule form is added which may be conveniently used in recording observations.

As the studies before us deal largely with the body and mind or the mental action of the brain, chapters will be devoted to the observation of mental expression and movement. This leads me to speak of the differences between signs which indicate general brain status, its health and power on the one hand, and mental expression on the other.

Case 6. A boy well made, healthy, and well grown in body, head, and features: his movements are quick and exact, he turns his eyes towards objects steadily and

imitates movements well, while his speech is good.
His body and brain appear well made and active. On
testing his mental ability it appeared that, though he
could count coins, he was not able to add their value or
calculate the change : he could read and write, but both
slowly and badly. The boy's brain was good enough
for the action and general activities of life and labour,
but the purely mental processes were performed very
indifferently.

The general conditions of make and power of brain
are ascertained by observation of the "nerve-signs,"
which are movements, action, balance, gestures, or other
motor acts ; they may be normal or below the normal.
Mental signs are mainly obtained in speech, expression
of judgment in making a choice, memory.

You will often find that modes of mental action,
whether good or faulty, correspond to the manner of
movement and action.

The child who, when spoken to, suddenly goes
through a number of extra-movements, excited but not
controlled by the spoken word, is liable, at the same
time, to mental confusion and may make some absurd
mental error.

Case 7. A boy whose eyes are wandering every-
where, with the head moving and the fingers twitching,
is asked to say what he knows about King Charles I.,
and replies that he had his head cut off at the battle of
Waterloo. Such mental confusion often accompanies

excessive nervous movements, and its removal may be helped by good physical training.

I shall not speak of Mind, Consciousness, Feeling, Will, and Judgment as something implanted in the body, — that is apart from and outside the scope of this work, — but I shall describe for you, as clearly as possible, in detail, with examples, all the points we can observe as indicating mental action in the brain, and analyse many modes of action and some verbal expressions, showing facts and faults in mental action.

Childhood presents so many varieties, that to deal with the subject concisely and in form convenient for study, it will be necessary to present certain classes and groups of children as we find them in the child population. Children may be classed as mentally bright or dull, as weak and delicate or nervous ; that is, according to certain difficulties we find in them: again, they may be grouped according to points seen in them, as quick and exact in all movements or slow in response and inexact in imitation ; as ill-proportioned in head and features, as over-mobile or motionless, or as deaf and of defective sight.

In an elementary school I saw 447 boys and 445 girls, of whom the teachers reported 41 boys and 23 girls as dull or backward pupils. Of these dull children only 6 boys and 11 girls were free of all faults that could be seen in the body and in action. Twenty-nine of these boys and 8 of these girls, found to be dull

at lessons, showed "abnormal nerve-signs," or indications of brain-disorderliness — slouching, listlessness,
inaccuracy in action and in looking, — points that
may generally be removed by good physical training,
whereupon improved mental action would probably
follow.   There were in all, 83 boys and 30 girls
grouped, as presenting these nerve-signs, showing how
much that school needed more attention to physical
training.

The method of observing what may be seen in each
child, and then grouping the children, according to the
points seen in them, may give much useful information.   The group "nerve-cases" was more than two
per cent above the average in this school.

A knowledge of the signs of the condition of the
brain will also be useful.   I have seen a young woman,
who presented the complete type of nervous exhaustion, standing before her class, truly an object for
sympathy, but a bad impression must have been produced thereby upon the pupils.

Let me present to you a report of what was seen at
a high-class school I was invited to visit.

Third class.   Twenty-nine boys present at a lecture
on geometry, 2.30 o'clock.   The lesson proceeded as
usual.   I observed the boys during the lecture, first
from the master's desk, afterwards from a side-table,
so as to get a good profile view.

This group of boys appeared generally healthy and

well. As I looked at each boy at his desk, eight of them attracted my attention : —

A, B. Two used spectacles.

C, D. Two did not use spectacles, but appeared to be short-sighted.

E, F. Two showed some developmental defects.

G, H. Two appeared somewhat exhausted in the nerve-system, and are likely to be subject to headaches; this is probably not a temporary condition.

No detailed examination of individual boys was made, but the grounds of the opinion given in the cases of E, F and G, H may be stated. E, F showed no signs of brain-exhaustion or of headaches. The following signs of defective development are probably of long standing, or from birth : —

Case 8. E. One of the biggest boys in the class; he must weigh heavy, and speaks with a loud voice. As signs of defective development I observed that the ears were ill-shapen, the head too round in form and wanting in characteristic points. As a sign of defect (probably permanent) in the nerve-system, there was excessive and coarse action of the muscles in the forehead, causing horizontal and vertical furrows. Evidence that he was not exhausted was seen in the symmetry of nerve-muscular action on the two sides of the body. It was observed that the over-muscular action of the face lessened as the lecture proceeded. He lost places in class.

Case 9. F. A small boy with a badly shapen head, though it was not small; this may have been due to rickets in early life. As to the nerve-system, he was too mobile, and there was a little over-action of the frontal muscles. He was distinctly fidgety or playful, and lost places in class.

Case 10. G. A boy of fair complexion, with light hair, rather under the average size, but placed second in class. The following signs of nerve-exhaustion were seen : too little general mobility in the limbs and in the mobile features of the face, producing a dull expression; in the forehead, however, there were fine horizontal lines or furrows, due to recurrent over-action of the frontal muscles. A further sign of exhaustion and probable liability to headaches was observed in marked fulness under the eyes. No signs of developmental defects were apparent.

Case 11. H. A boy of fair complexion, with light hair, placed twenty-fourth in the class; he lost places. The signs of nerve-exhaustion were: over-mobility; the arms were several times thrown about, often with the left hand clenched; he was decidedly fidgety. There was fulness under each eye, indicating that probably he is a sufferer from headaches. In addition, a slight sign of developmental defect was seen; the left ear was ill-formed.

Examples might easily be multiplied.

Of all the points to be indicated for your use in the observation and description of children, the " nerve-signs " will, I am sure, prove to be the most important and interesting, because it is the movements and balance, the gestures, action, and response, observed in the child that indicate or express his brain state. Here we have some new work, and these signs will, I hope, be of interest to you, because each depends upon the mode of action of some piece of the brain at the time you make your observation. Such signs of brain-disorderliness are much associated with the causes of mental dulness; as soon as the teacher recognises this, he will try, by further physical training, to improve the child in each aspect, and remove the signs of motor and mental disorder one by one.

CHAPTER II

The Body of the Child, its Construction and Growth

A BRIEF sketch of the infant will be useful to a full understanding of the development of the brain, as it quickly acquires some of those characters which give the child capacity for mental life.

The infant at birth weighs from seven to ten pounds.

	Male	Female
Average height or length in inches	19.34	18.98
Average weight in pounds	7.55	7.23
Average girth of chest in inches	13.25	12.65
Average circumference of head in inches . . .	13.95	13.57

The head of the infant differs in many particulars from that of the child of school age, and these are important to the proper understanding of its growth and some of the later defects. The bones of the skull are very thin, the size of the head very nearly corresponds with that of the brain which it contains; the bones are not united at their edges to form a rigid bony case as in the adult, but are separate at their margins so as to be movable on one another; this allows for a rapid increase in the size of the head as the brain grows. The size of the head is of interest, for small-headed infants are less likely to live; the brain is the principal seat of vitality. The corners of four of the bones are incomplete towards the top of the head, thus leaving an open space, called the soft spot or fontanelle, covered by a membrane and the scalp, where there is no bone; here the brain may be felt pulsating and swelling up when the infant cries.

The nose of the young infant is but little developed, and is flat and sunken in comparison with that of an older child.

At nine months old the fontanelle can still be felt, the head is still open and growing fast, it measures about $17\frac{1}{2}$ inches in circumference; at twelve months, 19 inches; and at seven years, 20 to 21 inches. You must not, however, expect always to find the head as large as here given, even in healthy children; but after three years old a circumference of 19 inches is too small.

Teething usually begins at the seventh or eighth month, the lower front teeth being the first to appear, then the corresponding ones in the upper jaw; the sharp-pointed canines come through at about the eighteenth month, and the others follow till the full number of twenty milk teeth appear, which is accomplished during the second year. At the age of six or seven years children begin to lose their first teeth,

c

and the permanent ones appear. It is hardly necessary to say that children's teeth should be kept carefully clean at all ages.

TABLE I. — OF DENTITION PERIODS

Temporary Set or Milk Teeth

First Group — Two lower central incisors appear .   6th to 8th month

Second Group — Four upper incisors appear . .   8th to 10th   "

Third Group — Lower lateral incisors, upper and
lower front molars, appear . . . .   12th to 14th   "

Fourth Group — Canines, upper usually first, appear   18th to 20th   "

Fifth Group — Posterior molars appear . . . .   2 years to 2½ years

	Molars	Canines	Incisors	
Full Set { Upper	2-2	1-1	2-2 }	20
Lower	2-2	1-1	2-2 }	

Permanent Teeth

Molars, first . . . . . . appear at . . . .   6 years

Incisors, central . . . . .   "   . . . . 7 "

 "   lateral . . . . .   "   . . . . 8 "

Bicuspids, anterior . . .   "   . . . . 9 "

 "   posterior . . . .   "   . . . . 10 "

Canines . . . .   "   . . . . . 11 to 12 "

Molars, second . . . . .   "   . . . . . 12 to 13 "

 "   third . . . . . .   "   . . . . . 17 to 25 "

	Molars	Bicuspids	Canines	Incisors	
Full Set { Upper	3-3	2-2	1-1	2-2 }	32
Lower	3-3	2-2	1-1	2-2 }	

We are now mainly concerned with the child of
school age; the head has grown rapidly since infancy
and should present neither ridges nor lumps, and the
brain has attained within a little of its full weight.

See Table V. The head has acquired a distinctive shape, expanding from the base at the level of the ears, its widest diameter being behind the situation of the ears, but with good expanse of forehead. The head contains the bony skull, the upper part of which forms the brain-case. The lower jaw is the only part of the skull that can move separately from the rest. This bone is jointed on to the skull; it is depressed when the teeth are separated, and brought up again by the muscles when the mouth is closed; the lower jaw can be moved up and down as well as laterally in mastication. The eyeballs are set in their sockets or cavities in the skull, called the orbits, resting among the fatty tissue which supports them. The movements of the eyes are produced by small muscles attached to the eyeball and arising from the walls of the orbit. These muscles are supplied by three different pairs of nerves from the brain. If the fat in the orbit be diminished in quantity, the eyeball sinks further into the orbit; if it receives more blood, it swells up and pushes the eyeball more forward. The coloured portion of the eye is called the iris; it is a muscular curtain with a hole in the centre which appears black : this aperture is called the pupil, and may contract or become very large. In description we must not confuse the eyeballs with the eyelids, which frame the openings for the eyes.

The face consists of the soft parts which lie in

front of the skull; under the skin there is a layer of
fat, and muscles passing in various directions which,
being attached to the skin, move it and produce the
expression of the face. A circular muscle surrounds
each of the openings of the face: the circular muscle
around each eye-opening is called the orbicularis
oculi; when it contracts, the eyelids are closed: the
mouth is closed in the same way. These muscles,
when stimulated by the nerves from the brain, move
the face, as will be explained in the next chapter.

Two pairs of muscles in the forehead are of special
interest to us: the frontal muscles are placed vertically and by their contraction raise the eyebrows
and produce horizontal creases in the skin of the
forehead; the corrugators are two small muscles,
placed in a horizontal position in the middle part of
the forehead which, when they contract, draw the
eyebrows together, producing vertical creases in the
mid-frontal region.

Two pairs of muscles seen in the face are concerned
in mastication, rather than with expression: these are
called the masseters — they are situated about the
angle of the jaw on either side; and the temporals,
which are placed at the side of the head, in those
parts called the temples. If you strongly clench your
teeth, you will feel these muscles become hard as they
contract and swell out. All these structures which
make up what is called the face are supplied with

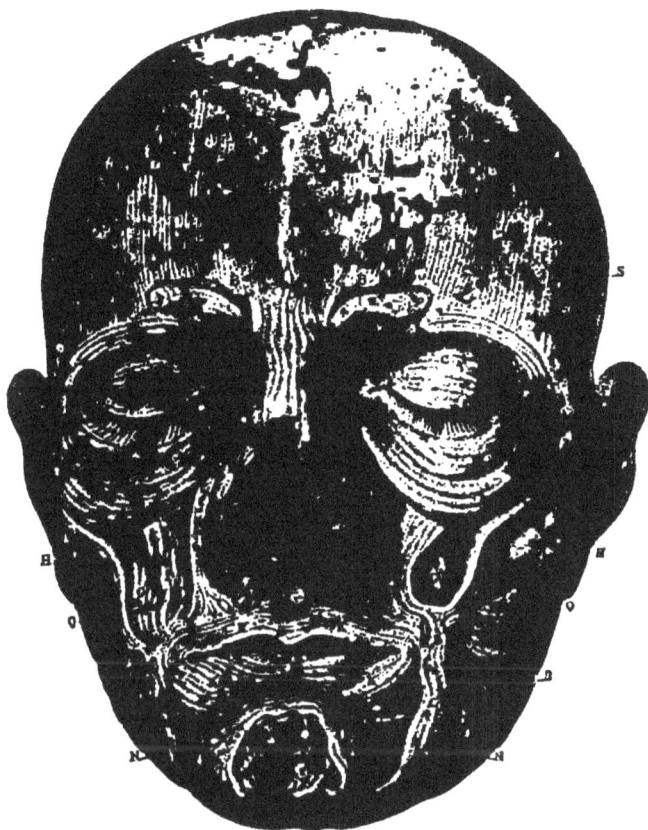

Fig. 1. — MUSCLES OF FACIAL EXPRESSION. — From Sir Charles Bell's *Anatomy and Philosophy of Expression*, Third Edition (Bohn Library).

AA   The frontal muscle.

BB   The corrugator muscle. It is inserted into the integument under the eyebrow. It lies nearly transversely, and its office is to knit and draw the eyebrows together.

CC   The circular muscle of the eyelids (orbicularis palpebrarum).

DEL Muscles moving the nostrils.

KK   The circular muscle of the mouth and lips. Its office is to close the lips; in excessive action it produces pouting.

HH   The zygomatic muscle. It is inserted at the angle of the mouth; by its action its widens the mouth, as in grinning.

NN   Depressor labiorum. It depresses the angles of the mouth; other muscles of expression are also represented.

blood-vessels, and the quantity of blood in them is also under brain control, through a nerve called the sympathetic. When much blood rushes to the face, the child is said to blush; when the sympathetic nerve allows but little blood to pass into it, the face is pale.

The openings for the eyes (palpebral fissures) are placed between the upper and the lower eyelids; the line joining the angles of the openings is horizontal.

The nose has been referred to as a feature in the face. It is necessary to understand its importance as the proper entrance for the air breathed; a free entrance of air by the nose is important to the child, and a knowledge of some points in the structure of the nose, throat, and organ of hearing is necessary to our purpose. Air entering by the nose passes above the hard and soft palate to the back of the throat, where a tube (eustachian) leads air into the portion of the ear which is concerned in hearing. If there is any obstruction to this free entrance of air, the child becomes deaf or dull of hearing. The nose is the proper way of entrance and exit for the air breathed, and the child should be able to breathe easily with the mouth closed and the lips together. If the child cannot breathe thus, but habitually keeps the lips parted, there is probably something wrong with the throat or nose. Such habitual mouth-breathing is very important; mouth-breathers need medical examination.

The external ears should be alike in form, and stand out but slightly from the head. The external ear con-
sists of parts each of which should be present: the rim or margin curls over slightly; in front of this is the pleat of the ear (antehelix) jutting out in front, and you will find it is thrust forward from the back; the lobe or drooping portion of the ear should come below the point of attach-ment to the head.

The trunk or body has a bony frame-work, of which the spine is the main prop or support. The spine consists of a number of small bones, united

Fig. 2.—BONES OF THE SPINE, CHEST, SHOULDER, ARM, AND HAND.— From Sir Charles Bell's work on *The Hand.*

by pads of cartilage or soft material, which allow of a certain amount of movement in the column formed

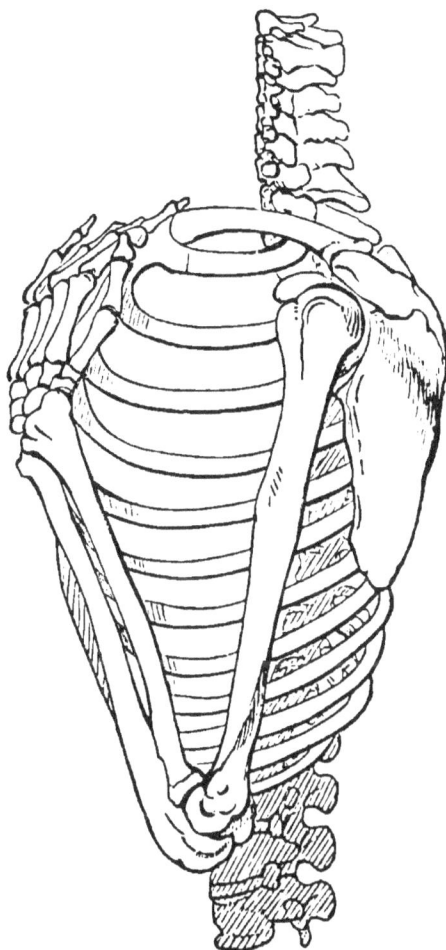

by the bones, so that the spine can be bent to some degree forwards and backwards or laterally. The skull is jointed to the top of this column.

The ribs are attached to the spine behind and to the breast bone in front, forming the walls of the chest.

The chest and the important organs, the heart and the lungs, which it contains, grow as the child grows. The average chest girth for children at various ages is given in Table IV. It is very important that the chest should be free to move in breathing: it should never be compressed by the dress.

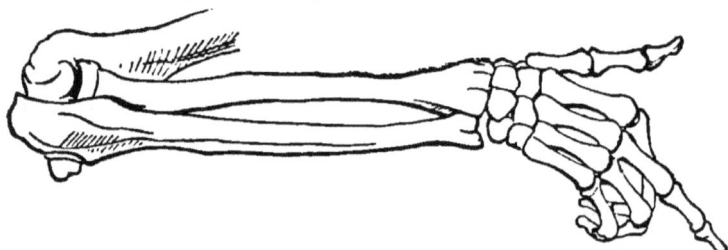

Fig. 3.—THE RADIUS AND ULNA.—In this sketch, the upper bone of the forearm is the radius, and in revolving on the lower bone, the ulna, it carries the hand with it. — C. Bell.

The arm or upper extremity consists of the blade bone placed over the back of the trunk; the collar bone stretches horizontally from the blade bone to the breast bone, and helps to keep it in its proper place; the arm is hung from this blade bone. The upper arm contains the bone called the humerus jointed at the shoulder to the blade bone. The forearm has two bones — the radius on the outer or thumb side, and the ulna on the inner side: these two bones are jointed

to the humerus at the elbow, and allow of two kinds
of movement. The elbow can be bent or, as we say,
flexed, and it can be straightened or extended : a rotatory movement or half a circle can also be performed
at the elbow. When the palm of the hand is brought
forward or laid upward, the forearm is said to be
supine, and this movement is called supination ; when
the back of the hand is brought forward, the movement
is called pronation. This rotatory action at the elbow
is due to movements of the radius on the humerus.

The wrist is composed of eight small bones, and
this joint allows of movements in all directions.

The hand has four fingers and a thumb, spoken
of collectively as the digits; these are united to five
bones, which form the palm of the hand and are
jointed at the wrist. The palm of the hand can be
moved at the wrist in flexion or extension as well
as laterally; it can also be contracted or screwed up
by bringing the bones together, so as to form the
hand like a cone. The digits can be flexed or extended, and they can be moved laterally.

These parts have been particularly mentioned because we are concerned with their separate movements.
When we look at a child we see these parts clothed
with their muscles and soft tissues, and covered with
skin; we observe the members, their form and proportions, and in some degree we judge of the development and state of nutrition of the child by such facts.

When examining a child, you should, if possible, weigh him and measure his height and chest girth, and also test sight and hearing. In taking a chest measurement let the child stand with his arms hanging by his sides, and make him count aloud the while to assure he is not holding in his breath. The measuring tape is then passed horizontally round the child on a level with the breast, and the number of inches in girth is recorded.

With growth from infancy the child becomes taller and increases in weight; this is shown in Table II., copied from Dr. Bowditch's article on the growth of children whom he measured in Boston.[1] It is here necessary to consider the boys and the girls separately and to compare them in age groups. It is interesting to note that, though at earlier ages the boys are on the average taller and heavier than the girls, yet at 13 to 14 years the girl outgrows the boy in each particular: after this age the boy again grows quicker to the stage of full development.

Children are best weighed in the morning in their ordinary indoor clothes, and measured in their stockings, without boots.

The average increase in height and weight is given in Table III., to which reference will again be made in Chapter X.

Growth, however, is not simply indicated by the

[1] See the *Annual Report of the State Board of Health, Massachusetts, 1877.*

height, chest measurement, and weight of the child; he may grow well developed or badly developed. A boy may be tall and heavy, yet not well developed in body and in features. It will be shown upon ample evidence from my observations, that defective physiognomy in make and proportioning of the features is apt to be accompanied by low brain-power with defective nutrition in after life. To study the general character of the development of the child's body the separate features of the face must be observed.

You want to know, as to the child's body, not only whether it is well grown and well developed for his age, but also whether he shows the indications of a well-nourished and healthy body in his physical life, as apart from his brain condition and mental power. Do not be guided in making your observations by indications of poverty, but satisfy yourself by what you see, that the child is not pale, thin, or delicate. The following points may help you : look at the face as to colour; do not mistake a fair complexion with light hair and blue eyes for paleness, or a dark complexion for its absence. Look also at the colour of the lips, and the colour seen through the finger-nails, which disappears upon pressure. A pale child may flush in the face, but such flushing is temporary. When you note the colour of the lips and skin, as signs of the general nutrition, observe also the hair and the eyes; when these are dark, it is owing to the amount of pigment in these structures, and then the skin is usually darker in its tint. Observe whether the colour comes and goes; such changes are due to the action of the nerve-system on the blood-vessels. If there be permanent paleness, it may be due to a poor state of the blood, called anæmia; then the child is out of health. A pale child may flush much. Defective colour may be due to ill feeding, to living in rooms badly ventilated, hot and close, or too dark.

The fulness, fatness, or plumpness of the child may not be alike all over the body. The face may be fairly full, while the limbs are thin. This is particularly the case in the nervous children, in whom the body weight may at times fall rapidly, dropping one or two pounds a week without any disease or even any failure of appetite; this is a condition in which a child commonly develops chorea (St. Vitus's dance); as the body weight drops, the face may continue to be the best nourished part, but the child is apt to become more infantile and over-mobile; this is specially apt to occur in girls. Weighing the child will add accuracy to your observations.

The eye may have a wrong focus. The eyeball is an optical instrument, which if properly arranged produces a clear picture of objects upon the retina, which is the sensitive layer at the back of the eye; it is something like the camera of the photographer, but its focus must be properly adjusted to produce clear sight: if the eye is out of focus, sight will be defective. There are two principal forms of badly built, badly proportioned eyes : —

1. The small flat eye. (Hypermetropia.)
2. The long eye, which causes short sight. (Myopia.)

The small flat eye is irregularly developed or proportioned at birth, the condition is congenital; it is undersized and the condition is often inherited. It does not produce clear pictures on the retina, and the focussing apparatus (muscle of accommodation) is strained, to produce clear vision of the letters in a book. This may lead to headaches or to squinting. Squinting is usually due to the eye being small and flat; such children, when old enough, should be provided with proper spectacles, and they should always use them when reading or writing.

The eye too long from front to back leads to such bad focussing that vision is indistinct and the child near-sighted. This condition is not found at birth, though the tendency to short sight may be inherited; it usually develops during school life, and is in part preventable by the use of glasses and attention to the position of the child when at work. Do not let children bend over their desks; still, remember that the short-sighted child cannot sit up and see his book on a flat desk. To save children from becoming short-sighted, prevent them from using their eyes too long and too closely on near objects. The boy should sit up well, with his head upright and his eyes at least twelve

inches from his book ; the desk should have a sloping
top, and the seat must be properly adjusted to his
height : books of bad type should always be avoided,
and the light should be sufficient, especially at night.

Each child should be tested as to sight when he
enters the school and at least once a year afterwards.
A set of printed type should be provided for the purpose : such are published, and arranged as to the size
of the letters so that with clear vision each line can be
seen at the distance named on the sheet; this should
be hung on the wall in a good light.   A child, standing
at the proper distance, should be able to read the letters
readily : test each eye separately, covering the other
with a card in front of it; if the child cannot thus
see the letters with each eye, there is some defect of
sight.

Again : let the child stand and look at a small coin
held before his face two feet from his nose ; if you see
that his eyes then turn inwards with the appearance of
a slight temporary cast or squint, he probably has flat
eyes (hypermetropia) and requires convex glasses.

You may test hearing by your watch or by your
voice.   In using your watch ascertain previously how
far from the head it can be heard by persons with good
hearing ; use a measuring tape, holding one end against
the ear and the other at the watch.   Direct the child
to close his eyes, and hold a sheet of paper or a fan to
prevent him from seeing the watch, while you make

him close the opening of the other ear, which you are not testing. Carry your watch to different distances from the side of his head, square with it, not in front of him. When he says he hears the watch, note the distance, move it to a further distance, and then back again to the former place, and see if he adheres to what he said before: test him thus several times and examine each ear separately, noting the greatest distance of hearing with each ear.

TABLE II.

SHOWING AVERAGE HEIGHTS AND WEIGHTS OF BOSTON SCHOOL
CHILDREN OF AMERICAN PARENTAGE

After Dr. Bowditch. See Annual Report of the State Board of Health, Massachusetts, 1877. Height taken without shoes ; weight in ordinary dress.

AGE LAST BIRTHDAY	BOYS		GIRLS	
	Inches	Pounds	Inches	Pounds
5 years	41.74	41.20	41.47	39.82
6 "	44.10	45.14	43.66	43.81
7 "	46.21	49.47	45.94	48.02
8 "	48.16	54.43	48.07	52.93
9 "	50.09	59.97	49.61	57.52
10 "	52.21	66.62	51.78	64.09
11 "	54.01	72.39	53.79	70.26
12 "	55.78	79.82	57.16	81.35
13 "	58.17	88.26	58.75	91.18
14 "	61.08	99.28	60.32	100.32
15 "	62.96	110.84	61.39	108.42
16 "	65.58	123.67	61.72	112.97
17 "	66.29	128.72	61.99	115.84
18 "	66.76	132.71	62.01	115.80

Testing with your voice has the advantage that if the child repeats what you say you know that he heard you. You should stand a distance of several yards from the child, while he keeps his eyes shut; he must not see your face, as he might read the sound from your lips; test first both ears together, then one at a time. An audible whisper may be heard much farther than the ticking of the watch; according to Mr. T. Mark Hovell, whispered speech should be heard at about twenty-five yards. To pronounce single words is better than to ask a question, which may be guessed at.

TABLE III.

SHOWING THE ANNUAL INCREASE IN HEIGHT AND WEIGHT

After Dr. Bowditch. *Vide ante.*

AGE LAST BIRTHDAY	Boys		Girls	
	Inches	Pounds	Inches	Pounds
5 years	—	—	—	—
6 "	2.36	3.94	2.19	3.99
7 "	2.11	4.33	2.2S	4.21
8 "	1.95	4.96	2.13	4.91
9 "	1.93	5.54	1.54	4.59
10 "	2.12	6.65	2.17	6.57
11 "	1.8o	5.77	2.01	6.17
12 "	1.77	7.43	3.37	11.09
13 "	2.39	8.44	1.59	9.83
14 "	2.91	11.02	1.57	9.14
15 "	1.8S	11.56	1.07	S.10
16 "	2.62	12.83	.33	4.55
17 "	.71	5.05	.27	2.87
18 "	.47	3.99	.02	0.04

TABLE IV.

SHOWING MEASUREMENTS OF CHEST GIRTH IN CHILDREN AT AGES CORRESPONDING

After Dr. C. Roberts' observations on the English artisan class.

AGE LAST BIRTHDAY	AVERAGE CHEST GIRTH IN INCHES	AGE LAST BIRTHDAY	AVERAGE CHEST GIRTH IN INCHES
5 years	21.40	13 years	25.24
6 "	21.68	14 "	26.28
7 "	22.54	15 "	27.51
8 "	23.09	16 "	28.97
9 "	23.79	17 "	29.38
10 "	24.08	18 "	30.07
11 "	24.34	19 "	30.56
12 "	24.93	20 "	30.86

TABLE V.

SHOWING THE AVERAGE WEIGHT OF THE BRAIN OF CHILDREN IN OUNCES AVOIRDUPOIS

After Dr. Boyd, as observed by him in 2030 cases, London. See Dr. Thurman's article on Weight of the Brain, *Journal of Mental Science*, 1866.

	MALES	FEMALES
New born	11.67	10.00
Under 3 months	17.42	15.94
From 3 to 6 months	21.30	19.76
From 6 to 12 months	27.40	25.70
From 1 to 2 years	33.25	29.80
From 2 to 4 years	38.70	34.97
From 4 to 7 years	40.23	40.11
From 7 to 14 years	45.96	49.78
From 14 to 20 years	48.54	43.94

D

CHAPTER III

WE now pass on to consider the brain itself, its functions, and the signs of its action. The brain is a part of the body hidden from our view, and enclosed in its bony case in the head. The brain of the child is carefully protected from injury, being surrounded by delicate membranes and a slight layer of fluid; it is well supplied with blood, which circulates and supplies it with needful nourishment.

The brain is a soft and delicate structure, seated in the brain-case, and carefully protected; it consists essentially of two kinds of material, the nerve-cells and the nerve-fibres. The nerve-cells are the makers of nerve-force when duly nourished; for their proper nutrition they need a good supply of blood in their vessels. A nerve-fibre passes off from each cell and conveys the force generated in it, which is then called a nerve-current; there are millions of such cells in the structure of the brain. When the nerve-force generated by a nerve-cell is carried by a fibre to a muscle, say in the face, or in the limbs, this nerve-current causes the muscle to contract or shorten, and

visible movement results; the movement being produced by the force sent from the nerve-cell. The
movement seen indicates to us the time and quantity
of the discharge of force from the nerve-cell: such
a movement is conveniently called a nerve-muscular
movement.

The substance of the brain is thus mainly made up
of groups of nerve-cells, many of which are connected
with one another by nerve-fibres, while many of them
are connected with the muscles of the body, and send
nerve-currents to them, thus causing the movements
of the face and limbs. The nerve-cell generates force
as the outcome of its nutrition, and may be compared
to a galvanic cell which generates electrical force as
the outcome of chemical action taking place in it.
The electrical force · formed in the galvanic cell may
be conducted to a distance by a wire, and if this end
be connected with a galvanometer, it may produce
movement of its needle at a distance from the battery. If several electrical cells be connected together
in series by means of wires, the force generated by one
cell is communicated to the next, and increases the
strength of the current circulating in the wire that
passes off from the battery; this force may be dis-
tributed to parts at a distance from its origin.

As time goes on, the strength of the battery will
run down, the chemical action in it lessens, the material in the battery is used up, and no more force is sent

out till the materials in the cell are renewed. Similarly: while the brain is giving out force, it must be replenished by nutrition, or it will run down and be less capable of producing energy after a short time; it will then need food and rest, and the stimulus which aids brain-nutrition.

I have spoken of the nerve-cells of the brain as being connected with one another, and with the muscles of the body, which produce movements of its parts. It must now be explained that there are other nerve-fibres which connect the organs of special sense — the eye and the ear, etc., and the skin all over the body — with the cells of the brain, and convey currents of force from these parts, respectively, to the cells of the brain; such nerve-fibres are called afferent, because they convey currents upwards to the nerve-system; in distinction from these, the fibres which convey currents from the nerve-cells to the muscles are called efferent. The fibres, which pass in both directions, are collected into bundles or strings, and are commonly called the nerves of the body; the in-going or afferent nerves convey stimuli to the brain, the outcoming or efferent nerves carry motor currents from the nerve-cells to the muscles.

Figure 4 may explain further what has just been said: the brain is represented by the shading as divided into areas *A*, *B*, *C*, *D*, *E*, which can act more or less independently; each area or section of

brain is represented as connected by nerve-fibres
with a muscle corresponding. Each section of brain
may receive a stimulus from the eye or the ear.
The representation is purely diagrammatic, for the

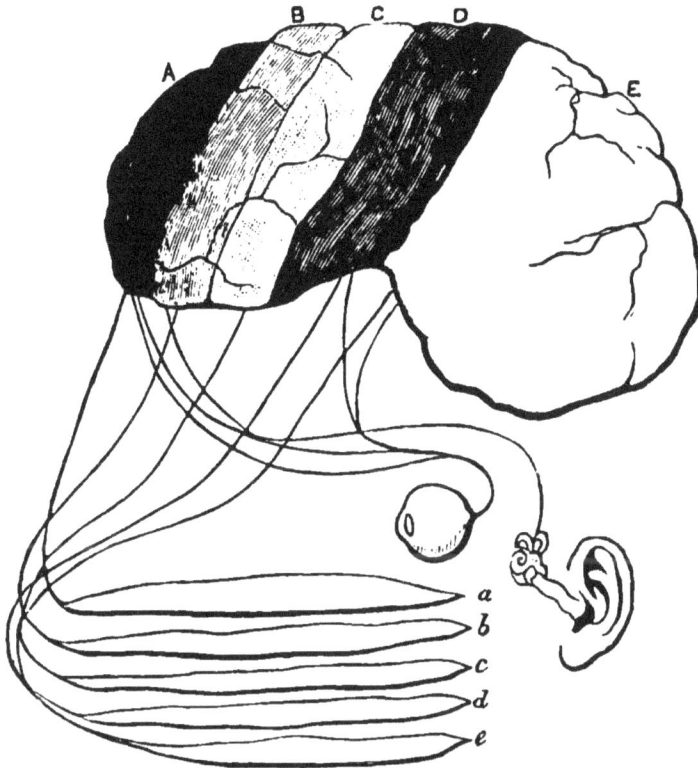

Fig. 4.— DIAGRAMMATIC REPRESENTATION OF THE BRAIN AND ITS
NERVES IN CONNECTION WITH THE EYE, THE EAR, AND THE
MUSCLES.

sake of clearness of description. The brain-areas
A, *B*, *C*, *D*, *E* each receive nerve-fibres carrying impressions from the eye and the ear, so that they
can separately be stimulated by sight and sound.

Fibres pass from each brain-area to the muscles *a*, *b*, *c*, *d*, *e*, respectively; when *A* is stimulated, the muscle *a* contracts; if the centre *E* be stimulated, the corresponding muscle *e* contracts, and so for each centre and muscle respectively; the muscle is the visible index of nerve-currents proceeding from its own centre. If we see the muscles *a*, *b*, contract at the same moment, that indicates that the centres *A*, *B* acted together.

If you see my arm move, you know this means that the muscles of my arm are contracting, and that this is due to currents of nerve-force passing out to them from certain nerve-cells by means of the efferent or motor nerves. Place an orange in front of a child; then you will see his head and eyes turn towards it, next his hand is moved over the orange, his fingers are closed over it, and it is seized. This series of movements is due to a series of nerve-currents passing from the nerve-cells to the muscles of the parts moving; this series of nerve-currents from the nerve-cells to the muscles follows the impression produced upon the brain, by the sight of the orange, or, by the afferent currents passing from the eye to the brain, and these are stimulated by the light reflected from the orange.

Many parts of the brain can act separately: every movement corresponds to the action of a certain portion of the nerve-system, or, as we call it, nerve-centre. It is probable that every movement indicates the discharge of force from a certain area of nerve-substance, and that such discharge of force necessitates not only a supply of good blood to that piece of nerve-tissue, but also that the nerve-tissue shall be stimulated by some force. Stimulation is necessary to movement as well as a supply of blood to the nerve-centre; sights and sounds are the more common stimuli to movements.

Important as the functions of the brain are, and much as we desire to study its action, there is only one way in which we can watch the effects of its working, and that is, by the movements which it produces in the parts of the body by its action on the muscles. All movements in the body are produced by the action of the nerve-system upon the muscles; this is very important to remember. Hence, we shall have much to say about movements, the outcome of movements, and mobile expression as signs of brain-action and the brain-condition.[1]

It may occur to you that, as much has been said by physiologists about the connection between the mind and the brain, we might study mental action as signs of brain-action. Let me make an assertion, and then support it by illustrations. *All expression of the action of mind is by movement, and the results of movement.* A child is at lessons, he repeats what

[1] See author's work on "Anatomy of Movement."

he has been taught, accompanied by gestures or movements; his speech is produced by the *movements* of his chest, larynx, and the parts used in articulation. The written exercise is the outcome of the *movements* of his hand acting upon the pen. His intelligence may be shown in a game, in the house he builds with his bricks, or in the paper-folding which he does so neatly with his fingers; in all such cases the signs of the action of mind are the *movements* produced by the brain.

The general condition of the nerve-system is expressed by motor signs — freshness, fatigue, irritability, may all be indicated to us by the movements of the child, the absence of movements, or by the attitudes or postures of the body, which depend upon motor action. Examples will be given in Chapter V.

The expression of the emotions is by the action of the brain upon the muscles of the body, and their contractions produce the signs which indicate to us what are called the emotions of the mind. We shall here study movements produced by the brain, not mind itself, in the child.

Look at a child before he wakes in the morning. The body is quiet; if you raise his hand gently, it falls lifeless — no muscular energy is being expended. The body is motionless in full sleep, except for the movements of breathing, which are quiet, regular, uniform. If sleep is full and complete, on raising

the eyelids the pupils are seen to be very small or
contracted. The body and brain are in complete rest;
in a healthy, well-fed child the whole system is in the
state of quiet nutrition of organic life; no currents
are being generated by the brain in perfect, dreamless
sleep. As time goes on, you hear sounds in the house
which send currents from the child's ear to his brain;
we then see some movements of the limbs — the
elbows, wrists, and fingers move. Soon all is seen to
be quiet again in the limbs — sleep continues, and
the brain rests and grows without expending force.
As sounds grow stronger in the house, and the light
pours in between the opened curtains, you may again
see movements in the limbs, and the eyelids open; the
pupils now dilate; the brain becomes active, indicated
by movements in the limbs and face, as the child sits
up. Nerve-currents are now passing from the brain
to the muscles. Before school he is full of movement;
limbs, fingers, head, eyes, are all moving, owing to spontaneous brain-activity. As he stands in his place, and
the teacher calls for attention, we see him still and
quiet (or at least that is desired), and the teacher tries
to control his brain-action under instruction. Spontaneous brain-action will be shown to be the basis
upon which you work in producing mental aptitude;
it must be coördinated or regulated, but so as not to
destroy spontaneity.

Two circumstances are necessary in order that a

nerve-centre may produce action of the muscles and
movement, — it must be nourished by good blood, and
it must receive some stimulus. This gives us the clue
as to how we must act upon the brain of the child :
there are two ways, — by feeding it and by *stimulating
it through the organs of sense.* Brains do not grow
by feeding only; they must be impressed or stimulated from without; hence the importance of good
education as an aid to brain-development. Feeding
the child often lessens spontaneous movements, when
they are in excess ; fresh air may have a similar effect ;
various modes of stimulating a child through the eye
and ear may control spontaneous movements, but these
must be used with due caution. Do not stop a child's
movements unless you know why you do so. You should
no more wantonly arrest a child's movements without due cause than throw a stone at an animal without
cause, or destroy a flower because you do not see any
use in it. This should be known by those who con-
fine the hands and feet of little infants under bulky and
cumbersome clothes. Children should have their hands
free, and not carry bags and books, and should not
be compelled to stand in class with their hands behind
them.

Common observation of a healthy young infant
shows abundant spontaneous movement in all parts
of the body while he is awake. Look at a well-nourished baby, say seven days old, as he lies on his nurse's

lap, unfettered by clothes. Movements are seen in the limbs, especially in the fingers and toes; the movements are slower than most of those seen in adults, and are apparently spontaneous and irregular, occurring in no special order, uncontrolled by external stimulation, and are not directly useful to the child. A short period of wakefulness is, at this early age, usually followed by sleep, indicated by subsidence of all movements except those of breathing, and the eyelids are closed.

The movements of the chest in breathing are established at birth, and continue without interruption. The child cries when cold, and when food has been withheld more than two hours. Contact of an object with the lips stimulates the movements of sucking; a strong light causes closure of the eyelids; and if the eyelid be raised, the pupils are contracted by the light. In an infant a few hours old, the attempt to straighten the elbow, when flexed, may be strongly resisted.

Spontaneous movements may likewise be seen in young animals. Charles Darwin has shown that in young seedling plants the root, the seedling leaves, and the head of the plant move much, as growth takes place, though the movement is slow. This is due to unequal growth of the cells of which the young plant is built up.

Spontaneous movements, thus universal at birth, must have some important signification; they do not appear to produce any direct effect upon the body of the infant and do not supply him with food or minister to his wants.

Each movement seen corresponds to action in a nerve-centre of the brain; the mass of movements corresponds to a mass of nerve-centres in action. Further, these movements, as far as we can see, are not at birth controlled through the senses. We conclude that in the very young infant the brain-centres act separately and independent of special stimulation, if he is healthy, well made, and well nourished. It may be said that at birth the infant does not show the faculties of mind, because we do not see that he is controlled through the senses by sight and by sound: his hands do not move towards objects placed within his field of vision.

When a month old, movements appear in the face, first about the mouth, later in the forehead. The limbs move with more force, they are moved in a greater degree, and begin to effect some mechanical results : an object placed in the hand is grasped by the fingers, and movements of the elbow carry the object to the mouth, but soon spontaneous movements return, the fingers open, and the object falls from the hand.

When the infant is three months old, we may observe some control of movements through the senses, and the head may turn towards a bright light; still we do not see the hand move straight towards an object within the field of vision, and when a part of the body is irritated the hand does not move towards it. I have known a child in whom one leg was irritated, and the hand was not moved to scratch it, but the other leg moved up, and did so with the foot. Spontaneous movement remains as a marked character at this age, but sight of a bright object may temporarily arrest it; this is the earliest indication of a brain-faculty that may develop into the power of attention.

Later we see associated movements in such an act, as transferring an object from one hand to the other: as the muscles grow stronger the head is held up, when the body is supported, and the eyes are moved. At four or five months we find commencing signs of impressionability to stimulation through the senses; sound and the sight of objects begin to control and regulate the spontaneous movement.

At five months, further indications of the control of brain-action may be seen; the sight of a red box may momentarily stop all movements, and this may be followed in a few seconds by turning the head, eyes, and hands towards the object seen; that is called a coördinated movement; movement controlled through the eyes occurs after momentary arrest of spontaneous action in the brain.

At three years of age much change has taken place in the brain as the body has grown: the child runs and talks or chatters. Spontaneous movement continues to a great extent, but action controlled through the senses is established, complex actions are performed, an impression received at one time may be retained and lead to special action at a later period.

Case 12. A boy of three years went to sit on the bed of his mother, who was tired and ill. He played with some reins fastened to the end of the bedstead, which pleased him : next day he said to his mother, " You go and be nice ill; I play horses." A brain-impression had been retained (memory), leading to his action.

I dwell on the simple signs of brain-action in the infant, because they seem to afford a foundation for observation of the more complex functions of the brain of the child, as the processes of development or evolution proceed. The infant at the earliest ages does not walk or talk, or turn his head and eyes towards objects ; movements are not modified in any marked degree by the action of light or of sound. The infant's brain is, in some respects, less impressionable than that of the adult, and the impressions are less retained. During the early months of infant life movements are the only signs of mental development. Compare the action seen at five months with that seen at birth; spontaneous movement continues, but is capable of some control through the senses. It may be temporarily arrested by sight or sound, and this, after many repetitions, may be followed by new series of movements, occurring upon less and less stimulation, and with increasing quickness and accuracy, as time goes on. We infer a corresponding change in the nerve-centres or parts of the brain: it appears that, at birth, they act slowly and independently of one another, as far as we know without any order in their acting — and, at this time, this action is not determined through the senses. At the age of five months movement may be temporarily suspended, and during the time when no (efferent or motor) currents are passing from the nerve-centres, they undergo some change, indicated subsequently by special combinations and series of movements, such as are commonly spoken of as commencing voluntary action.

This appears to be a great advance in the infant's brain-evolution.[1] When a year old, action well adapted by impressions received becomes very marked, and the child makes certain characteristic sounds on sight of certain objects; its spontaneous brain-action becomes more and more capable of coördination.

It appears that, whereas at birth the most marked character of the nerve-centres is the spontaneous action of individual loci of nerve-tissue, this spontaneity is not lost, but remains in advancing evolution as the foundation of so-called voluntary and intellectual action, becoming more controlled by circumstances. Aptitude for mental action appears to depend upon the capacity of nerve-cells for control through the senses, such impressions temporarily inhibiting their spontane-

[1] The Study of Cerebral Inhibition, "Brain," XLIII., published by The Macmillan Company.

ity and arranging them functionally for coördinated action. In the imbecile infant action does not show this spontaneous movement (microkinesis) in the normal degree; its nerve-centres are wanting in spontaneity, and later in capacity for coördination.

It is not my intention here to branch off into the study of physiological psychology, but it is quite possible to follow the apparent grouping of action in nerve-cells corresponding to many well-known modes of mental action. It may be shown that well-coordinated visible movements usually accompany well-controlled mental action, and that a spreading area of movement, not controlled, often accompanies mental confusion.

This spontaneous movement, slightly under control, is the character of healthy brain-action of children in the infant school, so that postures are less available as signs among these very young children, and spontaneous movement of their fingers is the normal action. The parts of the infant are then full of spontaneous movements; an exception is in the eye movements, which are not frequent in many cases. One of the endeavours of infant training should be to encourage eye movements, then to control them.

The most interesting signs of brain-condition are those which indicate to us the action of mind. One method of determining the signs of mind is to compare subjects, possessed of mind, with others, devoid of mind or nearly so. It will be granted that an infant at birth does not show well-marked signs of mind. The principal signs of mind are absent. An infant at birth may be said to possess none of the actual faculties of mind, although he is healthy; he may possess potentialities, but he shows no actual present signs of mind. An idiot, in growing up from infancy, does not show those signs, appropriate to his age, which indicate the functions of mind. The infant is said not to show actual signs of mind, though he may show potentialities. The infant at birth does not walk, talk, or turn his eyes and head towards a bright object within his field of vision; movements are not modified, in any marked degree, by the action of light or sound, except that the eyelids contract spasmodically in the light. The infant is, in some respects, less impressionable, and the impressions are less permanent than in the adult.

We say that the new-born infant does not give expression to the faculties of mind, because he does not present signs showing that he is impressed, even temporarily, by the sight of surrounding objects; he does not move his hands towards objects within his field of vision, and no movements indicate that he is impressed thereby. Reflexes of sight and sound are almost entirely absent. The muscles of the face are seen to act earliest in the lower zone, those about the mouth causing expression before those on the fore-

E

head (corrugators), which seem to be specially connected with expression of mind.

Now as to the child when four months old, we say that the attention is easily attracted, because the sight of objects and sounds causes the head to be moved (by reflex action) towards the light or source of sound. More than this, after the stimulus of the sight of an object has caused the head and eyes to be turned towards the object, the further stimulation of the brain may arrest all movement: this often happens when the attention is attracted. On the other hand, the sight of an object, after it has caused the head and eyes to be turned towards it, may increase the amount of movement in the child.

Playfulness is probably the result of spontaneous movement, together with an increased susceptibility to reflex action. The "playful child" has a happy face, owing to the healthy tone of the facial muscles and their nerve-centres.

The following observation of a child *eighteen months* old, illustrates how the dawning intellectuality is indicated by the complication and fitness of certain sets of movements : —

Case 13.´ The child, having both hands full of toys, desired to grasp a third ; he then put the toy from one hand quickly between his knees, and thus set one hand free to take hold of the desired object.

The following kinds of movements as signs of a

healthy infant brain deserve separate attention: movements following certain external agencies, light, sound; movements, the outcome of the essential (untrained) properties of the nerve-mechanism; movements resulting from (training) the acquired association of nerve-centres; movements, similar to those previously occurring from a like cause, showing retentiveness; movements in different areas, such as the small joints in contrast with large joints, or a different condition of movement of adjacent parts, such as the fingers. There may also be a symmetry of movements.

CHAPTER IV

OBSERVING THE CHILD: WHAT TO LOOK AT AND WHAT TO LOOK FOR

THE training of children and the improvement in methods of education have become so important that there has arisen a general demand for exact knowledge as to the conditions of children at home and in the school. It is necessary that we should learn to study children in a scientific manner, that we may know how best to train their development in mind and body, and take our part in aiding them to grow up with a sound constitution and full mental power.

The care of all classes of children is a very responsible work, demanding intelligent study and earnest care. It is not enough to study methods of education and school practice, the subjects to be taught and the methods of teaching them. Some knowledge of physiology is very useful; but it is also necessary to observe and study the children themselves individually, and collectively in groups, that we may know their individual tendencies, good and bad, and that their ever-varying condition may be at once perceived. We should see the signs of fatigue before exhaustion and irritability are obvious in imperfect lessons and bad behaviour; hence the necessity for an intelligent and precise knowledge of children enabling us to detect early signs of failure of strength and to classify them for the purpose of study.

It seems to me very desirable, if not essential to the proper study of children, that we should form a judgment by the signs which we observe, not by the answers to questions put to the child as to his thoughts and respecting health. I seldom ask a child if he has a headache, but often look for the signs of healthy brain strength and activity ; or of exhaustion, and direct indications of headache. Such observations may be made by any one who is in personal contact with children, by the mother among her children, or the teacher in the schoolroom.

Let me give a few examples. At an elementary school I visited the girls in its highest standard, or grade, in company with some friends, and asked the teacher to point out, unknown to the children, those who gave most trouble. Among them were two small, but well-made children—the nerve-system in each was exhausted. Had this been known by those in authority, might not these children have been exempted from examination, and the teacher from the necessity to press them on, though still requiring their attendance at school ?

Case 14. In a high-class school, a boy presented a general good development, but his nerve-system was exhausted ; he had far too much movement, showing brain irritability. The master said he worked well, but his father often expressed his desire that the lad might do more work, and rise in the school quickly; the head-master wished the same. Here is a case where knowledge of a precise kind, possessed by the master, would necessarily put power in his hands to act for the boy's real good. On the other hand, where development is slightly defective, but nutrition good, it is for the child's benefit that he should not be excused from due work, except when knowledge shows that the work is harmful. Regular and appropriate work is essential to due brain development and healthy growth.

There are many points of view from which we may study children; many lines of thought which may be followed. The method I would urge upon you is that of systematic observation, — that which I want you to study is that which you actually see, apart from any inferences drawn from facts: it is essential, in scientific work, not to confuse what you see and what you believe to exist. Let us study the child as we see him, with the best powers of our mind, and careful earnest thought.

To see the child well you need a good light; do not touch him, but look without stating your purpose. It is desirable to prevent the child from looking straight at you, *i.e.* at your eyes; for this purpose fix the child's eyes by telling him to look at some small object held in your hand, such as a shilling. Then you proceed to observe the head and the physiognomy of the individual features and their parts, the facial condition and expression, the eye-movements and other points in action.

Let him hold out his hands in front, with the palms downwards, showing him the position for a moment; thus you can see how he responds to command and imitates your action, while you can observe the points described as " nerve-signs," indicating his brain status. Judging from the various points thus seen, and without asking questions or speaking to the children, it is easy to group their conditions in various classes thus : —

A. As to *Development* of the body and features.

B. As to the *Brain condition* indicated by nerve-signs.

C. As to *Nutrition* and health of body.

Such observations may give new knowledge for your use. Those who acquire the most practical knowledge of childhood will, in the end, acquire power and success in the work of education and training.

Here is a schedule form for use in describing systematically what you see in a child : three headings, *A*, *B*, *C*, group the classes of points to be looked for.

Under *A*, describe signs of development in the separate parts, and any special characteristics.

Under *B*, note nerve-signs in parts of the body.

Under *C*, the state of physical health and nutrition.

Under School Report the mental and general character is described ; and in the Report on the Child his mental and physical condition is briefly summarised.

SCHEDULE FOR REPORT ON A SCHOOL CHILD

Number.   *Name.*
  Age last birthday.   *Place in school.*

A. Body : Development, features, etc.
  Head.

   Face.
   Ears.
   Nose.
   Palate.
   Growth.

B. Nerve-signs : Postures, movements, action.
   Expression.
   General balance of body.

   Expression.
   O. Oculi.
   Eye-movements.
   Head-balance.
   Hands.

C. Physical health and Nutrition.

   School Report.

   Report on Child.

As you look at the child, bear in mind the normal or healthy type of development; fix in your mind an ideal of good form, so that your attention may be arrested by the sight of any point in form or action that is below the normal.

Now, as to what to look at : there is each part of the body named in the schedule and described in Chapter II.

The Head. — Look at the head full-face, carrying your eyes from ear to ear over the top of the head, following its curve and estimating its size ; again carry your eyes from one ear to the other in a horizontal line, looking first at the right ear and its parts, then at the right eye-opening, the bridge of the nose, the left eye-opening, and the ear. Looking at the profile, follow the bridge of the nose up the forehead, noting if it be nearly vertical, or slope backwards, then over the curve of the top of the head and down to the nape of the neck. You may thus inspect the head in its configuration and estimate its volume by inspection. Place your hand flat upon the child's head, with your fingers spread, and thus estimate its volume by feeling it, noticing its form and any lumps or ridges of bone. Then, if you think necessary, you can measure the head round with a tape. Measure carefully the greatest horizontal circumference round the forehead : take a transverse measurement from one ear-opening to the other over the top of the head ; and again from the bridge of the nose over the top of the head to a projection you will feel at the back of the head just above the nape of the neck; such measurements taken at intervals of a few months will enable you to appreciate growth and increase of volume of the head.

As you look at children, observing their form, you will see some with a shapely, well-moulded head of good size, while others are ill-shapen or small; the features may be well-cut or defective in form.

Physiognomy is defined by Lavater as "the art or science of discerning the character of the mind from the features of the face." Such modes of study include notice of such proportions of the head as the following: the height and width of the forehead, or its narrowness from temple to temple, and the shallowness from the hair margin to the eyebrows; the greatest circumference of the head, which is something like 21 inches at eight years old, the measurement from ear to ear over the vertex being about 12 inches. The greatest transverse diameter of the head in a child is behind the ears; and the outline of face and head as seen full-face should give the greatest transverse diameter high up, well above the cheek-bones in the part forming the brain-case. The facial angle is seen best in profile.

In estimating the volume of the head, first look at it; note its form, and not solely the circumference or other measurements. A further idea of its volume may be gained by placing your hand on the head with your fingers open. Heads may be too large or too small; the forehead may present a lump on each side, or a ridge down its centre ; it may be shallow from above downwards, or narrow laterally. These defects of the head are of great importance, often being accompanied with a tendency in the child to be thin, delicate, and dull : much depends upon how he is treated at home and in school.

At every possible opportunity observe the outline, form, and size of people's heads, paying special attention to the points mentioned ; study the physiognomy of children and persons known to you, and draw your own conclusion as to the value of your observations.

Study also well-selected art representations of the human figure, in rest and in action, and learn from them the rule of perfection. In some school-rooms, photographs, engravings, and casts of the best antique statues are to be seen. I wish it were so in all cases, that we might learn from those who have long observed the human body what is excellent in form and outline, as well as graceful in movement and attitude.

The Face. — Looking at different types of faces, we are at once struck with the fact that the passive appearance of some expresses intellectuality, while others are marked by inborn vulgarity, apart from any special mobile expression. Elements contributing to the low vulgar type are a narrow and receding forehead, a large, prominent under-jaw, thick lips, and a thick immobile make of skin. Such signs are, however, not to be trusted too far.

The features, separately, may be well made without being proportioned to one another or rising well from the surface of the face. If the openings for the eyes and mouth are small in proportion to the face, it imparts a blank look. The size of the jawbones gives an appearance of firmness to the physiognomy, while either the upper or lower jaw-bones may be too small. If the upper-jaw is too small, the cheeks at this part are too close together, the palate is often narrow, and the teeth overcrowded.

The Nose and the Palate are very noteworthy; they are described in Chapter II. As a sign of development or make of body the form of the bony palate is only second to the head in importance. The mouth should be noted, when at rest, as to its size. A small mouth is a defect, and often accompanies throat obstruction leading to mouth-breathing.

The Ears should be observed separately, noting their size and symmetry; see if they lie fairly against the head and that all parts are present in the ear as they are described in Chapter II.

The Growth of Body is estimated by the height and weight of the child as compared with the normal (see Table II.).

Passing from the observation of points indicating
development in the body, we have to consider the
nerve-signs, which indicate the make, status, and action
of the brain and nerve-system : these are mainly postures or attitudes of the body or action and movement of
its parts. Following the sub-headings of the Schedule,
look at the general balance of the body, the face, eyes,
head, and hands.

The General Balance of the body of the child, when
standing quietly, should be symmetrical, equal on the
two sides, so that the shoulders are at the same level
and the spine balanced straight ; while the feet are
equally planted on the ground with the knees straight.
When the arms are held out in front, symmetry should
be maintained in the equal height at which they are
placed with the elbows straight : no slouching or listless
attitude.

The Face and Expression. — The human face in its
expression and movements is a most accurate index of
the brain and of the nerve-changes in it, which correspond to the emotions, feelings, and thoughts.

When we look at a face, we may observe its form,
colour, and conditions of mobility. The general form
and outline of the face are largely determined by the
shape of the skull beneath. Either side of the face can
move separately; hence the necessity of observing
whether a facial expression is symmetrical.

The muscles that move the face are sufficiently ex-

plained in Chapter II.; their action in producing movement is caused by nerve-currents coming to them from
the brain.

The healthy normal face of a child is calm, without
wrinkling or puckering in the forehead, and is alike in
its action and expression on the two sides.

It is convenient, for the purpose of description, to
divide the face into three zones; the frontal above the
line of the eyebrows, with a middle zone separated from
the lower by a line at the level of the lower margin of
the orbits.

To observe each in turn, hold a sheet of paper with
one margin horizontal, leaving the forehead above the
eyebrows uncovered — this shows the upper zone; next
view only that part of the face which is below the lower
margin of the orbits, or sockets for the eyes, showing
the mouth, the greater part of the cheeks, and the
openings of the nose — this is the lower zone. Lastly
the middle zone may be demonstrated alone by holding
the horizontal margin of one sheet of paper so as to
cover all above the eyebrows, and another sheet so as
to cover all below the orbits, thus leaving to view the
eyebrows, the eyelids, and eyeballs, with the bridge of
the nose. By these methods you may readily examine
the symmetry of a face, both as regards form and
action, and you may also define the particular zone in
which any mode of expression is seen.

The greatest degree of expression is, I think, seen in

the frontal region, mainly produced by action of the frontal and corrugator muscles.

In looking at the mid-zone of the head and face, the observer's eye traverses it from ear to ear, noting these features, the palpebral fissures, and the tone of the large orbicularis oculi muscles, the bridge of the nose both in its bone and soft tissues, as well as the eyeballs and their movements.

Signs are given for each of the three zones.

There are some special movements in each of the facial zones worthy of notice. In the upper or frontal zone the movements are almost always symmetrical or equal on both sides; they may produce horizontal furrows, or vertical furrows with a drawing of the eyebrows together — the former is a movement not of an intellectual kind; the latter is often highly expressive of mental action.

In the middle zone the opening of the eyelids is usually equal on either side; we shall find that in this region we may have marked indications of exhaustion of brain-action.

The parts in the lower zone about the mouth move in eating and in speaking. The mouth can be widened, its angles may be drawn upwards or downwards, and the upper lip may be raised at a point a little within the angle, so as to uncover the canine tooth, as in sneering. Widening of the mouth is seen in laughter, when the angles are drawn some-

what upwards, so also, to a less degree, in smiling.
The circular muscle of the mouth contracts in closing the lips, and its action is excessive in pouting.

The Eye-movements are of great interest. In examining a child, notice whether the eyes follow accurately a small object you hold two or three feet
in front of his face, as you move it from side to
side, and up and down.

The two eyes move together, so that, when one
turns to the right, so does the other; or, when one
eye turns upwards, they both turn up equally. In
looking at near objects, say at 10 inches from the
face, the eyes turn slightly but equally towards one
another.

Movements of the eyes are not equally common
in all directions — more movements are horizontal
than vertical; in turning the eyes to the right or
left, there is no necessary movement of the eyelids;
the eyes turn towards objects, their muscles being
stimulated by brain-currents which are generated by
the sight of objects around. In observing movements
of the eyes, notice whether they are obviously guided
by the sight or sound of objects around, or whether
it be not so. Movements of the eyes, not controlled
as to their number and direction by obvious circumstances, must be looked upon as signs of nervousness. Irregular movements of the eyes are common
in children, and are very indicative of their brain-

condition : they may be looked upon as analogous to spontaneous twitchings of the fingers. In these wandering, irregular movements of the eyes we find an illustration of a common law, that excessive movement is often an indication of weakness, not of strength ; the same thing is seen in the twitching movements of nervous children.

Movements of the eyes in the vertical direction are accompanied by movements of the upper eyelids, and very often the eyes and head move upwards together.

The movements of the eyeballs are effected by small muscles attached to the eye and arising from the wall of the orbit; these small muscles are supplied by three different pairs of brain-nerves. The iris, or coloured portion of the eye, is a muscular curtain, with an aperture in its centre called the pupil, which may enlarge or contract. Light causes the pupil to contract; the pupil also contracts, when the eye is looking at near objects, dilating when looking into the distance. A widely dilated pupil may indicate a state of mental excitement; it is contracted in sleep.

The Head, its Postures and Movements. — It is convenient, for the purposes of description, to speak of three modes of movement of the head : *flexion* and *extension*, *i.e.* bending forwards and backwards, as in nodding ; *rotation* in a horizontal plane, the head re-

F

maining erect, but the face turning to the right or
the left side; *inclination*, *i.e.* lowering one or other
side of the head, so that the two ears are not on
the same level and the eyes not in the same horizontal plane — inclination is said to be towards that
side on which the ear is lowest. The only symmetrical movements of the head are those of nodding and bending back the head. In a strong and
healthy child the head is held erect unless something changes its posture. A slight sound may cause
rotation of the head; a slight condition of weakness
of the nerve-centres is indicated by drooping of the
head. The posture or balance of the head may indicate the brain-condition.

The simplest postures of the head are those called
flexion and extension; they involve equal action of
both sides of the brain. The weight of the head
makes it fall forward, if the muscles do not hold it
up; hence, as fatigue comes, and passes on to sleep,
the head may fall more and more forward, till it is
bowed on the breast. This bowed position of the
head indicates something about the condition of the
brain, but the posture is not solely caused by the
brain-action. Do not let children, when writing,
bend much over their desks — the face should be as
nearly vertical as may be, and as far as possible
removed from the horizontal. You may notice the
drooped head and the stooping and spiritless gait of

a tired man, as compared with that of the same individual when rested and refreshed. The head is
seen firmly upright in defiance, drooping in shame,
and held on one side in nervous girls.

The Hand. — The hand in its balance and movement
is second only to the face in importance as an index
of brain-action. In observing it for this purpose, the
hand should be held out free in front of the body,
not engaged in holding anything, but simply balanced,
as the brain controls the muscles. I have described
eight typical hand-postures : two of these will be given
among abnormal nerve-signs. When the hands are
held out to command, the average balance is with
both upper extremities horizontal on a level with the
shoulders, the hands turned palm downwards, the width
of the ˙chest apart, the elbows being quite straight.
The arm and the hand and its parts being all balanced
in the same plane, the palm of the hand spread flat,
and the fingers and thumb straight with the palm.

In observing a child, I say to him, " Put out your
hands with the palms downwards and spread the
fingers." The movements and balance of action in
the parts of the arm can thus be seen under favourable circumstances. A strong and healthy child, say
of five years old and upwards, will hold out his hands
fairly straight with the arm and shoulder ; the limbs
may not be held quite at the same level — the left is
often a little weaker and is held a little lower than the

right. The typical sign of strength is that the hand
be straight extended, as in Fig. 5, the fingers straight
with the metacarpal bones and the forearm and
shoulder; the palm of the hand, or metacarpus, straight,
not contracted laterally, as in the feeble hand (see Fig.
17); all parts are in the same horizontal plane; the

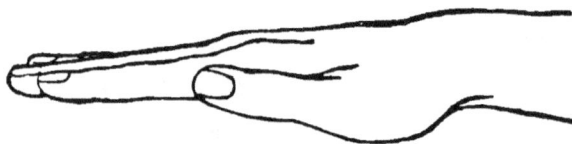

Fig. 5.—STRAIGHT HAND.

arms should be parallel to one another, straight at the
elbow and both on a level with the shoulder. A slight
deviation from this rather stiff and exactly balanced
position is not to be considered necessarily a departure
from health. However, the posture above described is
the standard of the normal, and indicates a robust, well-
balanced nerve-system.

CHAPTER V

PRINCIPLES OF METHODS OF OBSERVING AND DESCRIBING CHILDREN

CHILDREN may be studied in many ways. We may read about them and think about them; we may study the results of their work at school or the methods by which others teach and train them. We may study books on physiology which show how the circulation, digestion, and respiration are carried on. We may study the structure and uses of the organs of special sense, their connexion with the brain, and how they influence its action. All such studies are of value to you; still, there remains the question, " How may we, as individuals interested in children, best study them for ourselves ? "

In speaking of my own methods of examining and studying children, it is with the full acknowledgment that other means may be used; but it is my purpose to speak of what I have seen and of the methods employed in reporting on 100,000 children I have had opportunities of examining in 168 schools.

These methods I was gradually led to systemize in my own studies, and I have used them now for some

years. They are founded upon scientific and physiological principles, and necessitate observing individual
children and thinking about the facts observed. Such
a mode of study requires that facts shall be observed by
you, recorded and thought over; still be not discour-
aged; a little steady practice will make all easy, and
the effort will, I think, teach you much, give pleasant
study, and place a real power in your hands.

It will at once be obvious that the facts we are to
observe must be physical facts. We cannot directly
observe the action of the child's mind with our eyes
and ears; but we can observe the child's body, its
make, its movements, and the signs of its nutrition —
these can be seen and recorded in words; they can be
thought over and studied.

To observe children with success, we must learn
what to look at in an individual child, and how to describe what we see. To know how to describe what
is seen is almost as important, to our purposes, as to
know what to look for. Such descriptions aid our
memory; they enable us to compare observations, to
think about them, and to see their meaning.

The outward appearance of the body or the passive
expression has been studied from ancient times, and
much has been written on the subject. The laws of
form and the proportions of the body have been laid
down by many authorities who differ much among
themselves. Such studies have mostly been under-

taken from the philosophical and artistic points of view, rather than as a part of the study of mental physiology.

Much has been written on the subject of physiognomy that may interest you. Compare the writings of Lavater, and those who followed in his steps, with the later work of Sir Charles Bell on the " Philosophy and Anatomy of Expression." The knowledge and the methods of the two authors differ. Lavater described the size and form of the head of the man — he did not know the signs of brain-action; he observed the immobile signs — we shall see their significance presently. Sir Charles Bell described not only the anatomy of the brain and the nerve-system, and the muscles which produce movement; he showed that the brain by its action, as it sits hidden from view in the head, sends out currents of force to the muscles all over the body, producing those movements which we call mobile expression. Bell showed, further, that currents are constantly passing from the surface of the body and from the senses up to the brain, guiding and controlling its action.

We want to study the signs of brain-action. You will ask, What is the connexion between physiognomy and brain-action? As to the size of the head in connexion with the brain, it is certain that the brain can be no larger than the bony case which contains it ; further, the brain is often badly made when the head is badly shapen ; we shall see more about this further on. Experience shows that, when the head and features are badly shapen, the brain is often, but not necessarily, poorly developed. Defect in physiognomy and, in proportion, of the parts of the body, is often associated with mental dulness, but the occurrence of brain-disorderliness, indicated by abnormal nerve-signs (incoordination), is a more general and direct cause. It should then be an object, in training children, to remove their faulty nerve-signs or irregular or bad modes of action in movements, which are the direct indications of the brain-state. The most important signs of brain-action that we can observe are the movements which it produces in the body. It is by observing the action and attitudes of the child, that we find means of describing his brain-condition. The signs of brain-action, and the most valuable signs of its condition, are the movements and results of the movements which it produces in the parts of the body. It is of great importance clearly to understand the difference between the two modes of expression — passive immobile expression indicated by the size and proportions of the head and other parts, and the mobile expression or movement, which are the direct outcome of brain-action upon the muscles. The most important signs of brain-action are the movements, and results of the movements, which it produces, such as the postures and attitudes of the body, and speech : they are the direct outcome of brain-action, and can be observed and studied by all.

When I visit my country friend, he takes me to his stable and shows his horses, pointing out in each certain points of value for my admiration: in his hunter the height, sloping shoulder, small head, well-cut, straight legs, his clear eye; then he goes on to show the fine balance of his head, and when the horse is exercised, my friend points out the action seen in the movements of his limbs: we admire all these points and the well-groomed, fine, glossy coat. In the cart horse we look for more massive development and strength of limb and muscular growth. Again, in the farm he shows his bullocks, their small horns, straight backs, short legs, while pointing with pride to their fatness. In the corn-field he shows the number of large grains in each ear, the length of the straw and its cleanness : all points worth money.

In the nursery my friend shows me his "fine youngsters," but does not indicate the points of their hopefulness as well as he did the points in his animals.

In some reports on schools we are told the number of boys and girls in attendance, arranged in age-groups with the positions they hold in school — sometimes the boys are not divided from the girls. More strictly educational reports may indicate the number of dull, backward, and neglected children. All such accounts of childhood leave much to be desired : we need a census of the child-population ; we want to know the children as accurately as the farmer knows his horses, cattle, and corn. What principles, then, underlie the better methods of description? Individuals must be described; further, certain points in the individual should be described which may be compared in other individuals. Again: in describing his horse the farmer drew attention to the development and growth of the body in various points, then to his action in different movements, as in walking, trotting, galloping; he thus unconsciously explained something of the action of the animal's brain and nerve-system. These illustrations serve to show two principles that should be attended to in observing children. Look at their bodies, separate features and the limbs, as explained in Chapter II., and describe what is well made, and any badly made or faulty part.

The chapter on abnormal signs will help you to describe the defects in development and in action and expression.

Look also at the movements, the parts moving and the balance or attitudes, which indicate motor power and strength, and express brain-action.

The child is part of Nature's work; look at him as such, and study him as you study other living things. In short, I urge the scientific method, the methods of physical science, in place of relying on the meta-physical study of mind, when new knowledge and experience have to be acquired. I would urge you to the study of brain-action in producing the display of mind, and its causes, in place of confining your attention to metaphysical psychology : in saying this, I do not assume that this is new to you. The two methods differ, I think, principally in this: the psychologist proceeding to deal with most complex questions records complex results (mental states) of complex causes; the student of physical facts observes only what can be seen, reducing physical phenomena, that are complex, to their simplest elements, and notes their antecedents and sequents. The two methods may go side by side, they need not be considered as antagonistic; use such processes of study as give you the best results.

When a child is brought to a doctor for advice, he examines and observes him, he examines the body of the child and its various organs, taking notes of what he sees and hears. He forms an opinion of the pathology or real condition of the parts of the body by physical signs, then makes his diagnosis, and, after further considering the physical antecedents, which have probably brought about the conditions observed, he finally advises as to treatment. The friends of the child will also demand a prognosis, or opinion as to what is likely to happen in the future : this is often what is most urgently desired.

We shall have much to say hereafter about the signs of mobile expression, but before we pass away from the study of the body in its immobile or passive condition, a few words may be said as to the means of training the eye to recognise the perfect outline and form, and to observe any slight departures therefrom. For the purpose of training your eyes to appreciate perfections of form and accuracy of movement and balance, so that any deviations therefrom may be readily observed, use your powers of observation at every opportunity, observe your friends and acquaintances and all round you; specially observe children according to the rules laid down; try to form a general opinion in each case whether they be intelligent and well-bred children, then describe their form for yourselves as best you can, and fix those examples in your memory that are of high-class type; go into schools in poor districts, and study the less-well-born children. The types of perfection of form should be seen in art — they are seen in much of the antique and in some modern statuary; works of art may thus be useful to you. To study perfection and beauty of form you should contrast the most perfect with the least perfect. Examples of low development in contrast with more perfect productions will throw much light upon your studies; the contrast of marked perfection with imperfection throws each into greater relief and prominence. Leonardo da Vinci, we are told, searched for ugliness.

The head and face are parts of the body peculiarly characteristic of man, and here we see the greatest number of those signs which indicate to us the make of the individual and his condition. The head and face are also easily observed, and very interesting to study.

When studying expression in the head, as in other parts of the body, we must look to the conditions of its development, or size and form, and also to its movements and the postures which result from those movements. The title of Sir Charles Bell's first essay[1] is: "Of the Permanent Form of the Head and Face in contradistinction to Expression." He goes on to say: "A face may be beautiful in sleep, and a statue without expression may be highly beautiful; on the other hand, expression may give charm to a face the most ordinary. Hence it appears that our inquiry divides itself into the permanent form of the head and face, and the motion of the features, or the expression." Bell uses the term "expression" as confined to mobile modes of expression, and carefully distinguishes between them and conditions of development indicated by form. It seems probable, that the finer actions of the brain, in producing thoughts, may be trained by using good works of art. Form is probably more effectual for this purpose than shading and colour.

The Signs of Nutrition of the body and the brain are of the highest importance and interest. The first point I wish to insist on, is that nutrition may be expressed by (1) form or growth, and (2) by motion which is due to nutrition.

[1] *Op. cit.,* p. 21.

As evidence that motor signs, or movements and the results of movements, may express nutrition of brain, let us examine a few examples.

(1) In an ill-nourished infant spontaneous movement is much lessened, or the child may lie almost motionless instead of being constantly full of movement, while awake. The return of spontaneous movement is a sign of the improved nutrition.

(2) In a man after a severe illness, such as a fever, the tone of the voice is usually altered so that we can no longer recognise the individual by his voice; this motor sign, as well as the worn countenance, indicates the man's lowered nutrition. Returning health is shown by the patient "looking like himself," and "recovering his old voice."

(3) In a child seven years old emaciation and ill-nutrition, indicated by loss of weight, may be accompanied by St. Vitus's dance or finger twitching, which disappears when weight increases and nutrition is improved.

(4) A strong, well-nourished man is less fidgety than a weak one.

Now as to the expression of nutrition by form and growth. Proportions of growth often indicate conditions of nutrition.

A seedling pea-plant, if kept in a room with deficient light, is not well nourished, and the malnutrition is indicated by the small yellow leaves and the long white stem. That good nutrition has not occurred during the life of the plant is demonstrated by the fact that the plant, when dry, weighs less than the seed from which it grew. Here malnutrition is expressed by the relative growth of leaves and stem; the leaves being very small, the stem very long. In children we often see growth for a time occur in height without lateral development; then the proportions of growth change, and the child fattens.

It may possibly add some interest to our work, if I explain how my attention became directed to the study of postures as signs of brain-conditions. Having, during some years, given special study to the conditions of the nerve-system in children, I began to note the various postures presented by children, brought for examination, at the East London Children's Hospital, and from 1878 I kept notes of the spontaneous postures observed. The children were requested to hold out their hands, and the passive condition or posture of the hand was noted. At first it was difficult to describe the posture seen in precise language, though some were seen to be characteristic of certain nerve-conditions. In 1879, while visiting Florence. it struck me that the posture of the hands of the Venus de' Medici was exactly similar to the posture I had so often seen in nervous children. Later, at the British Museum, I saw the English Venus side by side with the Diana (Fig. 7), feminine coyness and nervous-

ness represented side by side with the expression of
energy and strength, and the contrast of the hand-
posture showed them to be in direct antithesis. While
looking at the marble hands, it became easy to describe
their postures in precise language. In the hands of
the nervous woman the wrist is slightly flexed or bent,
the knuckles are moderately extended back beyond the
straight line, the finger-joints being slightly bent. The
thumb is extended backwards, and somewhat drawn
away from the fingers. This posture I have called the

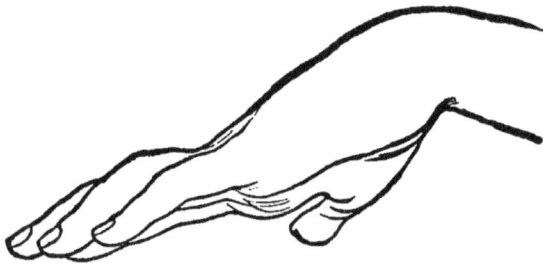

Fig. 6. — NERVOUS HAND.

"nervous hand"; it is that so commonly seen in weak,
excitable, nervous children, such as are hot-tempered
but affectionate, tooth-grinders, and very liable to recurrent headaches. I have before me the cast of a
hand carved by Canova, an art model of beautiful
workmanship. This hand represents exactly the nervous posture. Art often presents us with the expression of weakness in place of strength, beauty in place
of perfectness.

In the Diana of the British Museum we see the figure

of a strong, energetic woman. Our common experience tells us that it is such. Her right hand is lifted, and is engaged in holding a spear or dart, which she is about to hurl; this hand is, therefore, not available as a sign indicating the mental condition. The left hand, however, hangs down, and is free or unoccupied, and by its posture affords us evidence of the active or mentally energetic condition of the brain. The balance of the parts of the body indicates to us the balance of the action of the nerve-centres. This is the posture termed "the energetic hand " (Fig. 8).

The wrist is extended backwards, the fingers and thumb are flexed.

If we compare this energetic hand with the hand in the nervous posture, we see the former to be the direct antithesis of the latter. In the weak woman the hand is flexed at the wrist, the fingers and thumb bent back at the knuckles; in the strong woman the wrist is extended

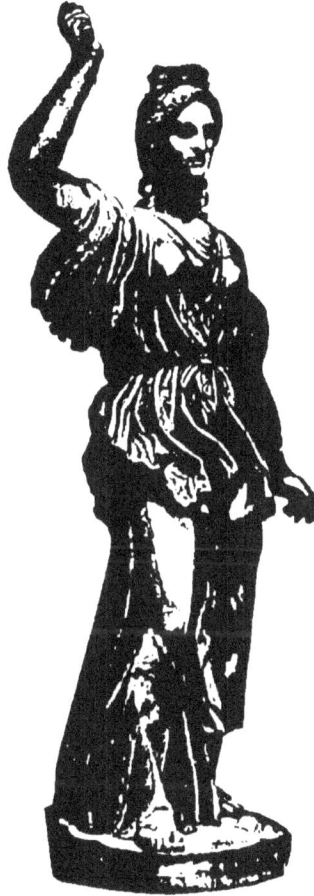

Fig. 7. — STATUE OF DIANA. British Museum.

G

backwards, and the digits are flexed. This is an example of one posture being the antithesis or direct opposite
of the other; Mr. C. Darwin made much use of the
principle of antithesis in his work on Expression.

I have described the straight extended hand as the
normal type, and two postures as deviations therefrom :
one, the energetic hand, a perfectly normal and health-
ful condition, the other the nervous hand, which indicates
weakness and excitability. An example of the energetic
hand in real life may often be seen in the attitude of

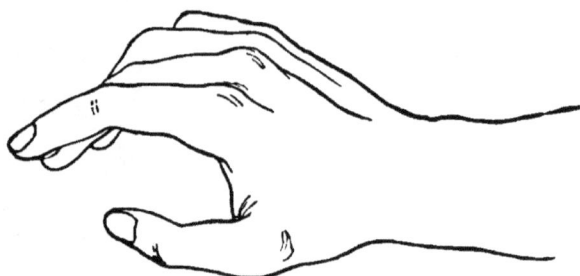

Fig. 8.—ENERGETIC HAND.

little children, say between three and four years old :
you call them to come to you, and show them something
they like ; they run with arms stretched out and hands
in the energetic posture, and wrist extended, and the
fingers slightly flexed.

An incident which happened the other day may
serve to illustrate the value of studying postures as
signs of the nerve-condition. I was asked to observe
some young people, and noticed three in whom the
hands, when held out free, showed the wrists flexed

with the knuckle-joints extended backwards. I immediately pointed out to the teacher that they showed some signs of nerve-muscular excitability; the correctness of this opinion I was afterwards able to confirm.

One of the first departures from the signs of perfect strength is the posture we are about to describe under the name of the "straight hand with the thumb drooped." This may commonly be observed in conditions of health, when fatigue or slight weakness occurs. It is similar to the straight hand, but the thumb, with

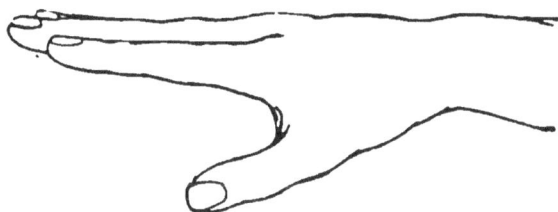

Fig. 9.—STRAIGHT HAND WITH THUMB DROOPED.

its metacarpal bone, falls slightly, thus approximating the latter towards the palm. I was once able to point out this sign to the head-master of a large school. I had looked over the lower classes of the school without noticing any unusual signs among the boys. When, however, we came to the first class, and these boys held out their hands, I observed that every boy, with two exceptions, held the hands straight, with the thumbs drooped. This class had recently been engaged in their annual examinations.

If you notice people's hands, you will often see

that early in the morning the hand is held quite
straight while in the latter part of the day the
thumb tends to droop. In such cases, food, and a
little rest, will usually restore the normal posture,
and this, the first sign of fatigue, will pass away.
This posture is, in fact, the first stage towards the
feeble hand, which I shall soon describe.

Figure 10 shows the natural position of the free
hand when at rest, as it may be seen hanging over
the side of a chair, or lying in the lap. The hand in

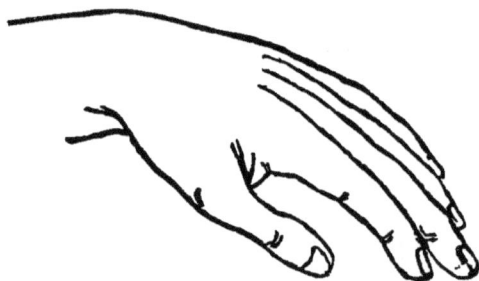

Fig. 10.—HAND IN REST.

rest is a natural position, with slight flexion of the
wrist and fingers, and slight arching of the metacarpus
or palm of the hand; it is also common in slight fatigue
without exhaustion, and may be seen in healthy sleep,
when no energizing nerve-currents are passing from
the brain to the muscles. If you are in doubt as to
whether a child is asleep, raise the arm by the wrist-
band and let the hand hang free; if the child be
asleep, the hand will assume the posture of rest.

The "feeble hand" is an exaggerated form of the

"hand in rest." The degree of flexion of all parts
is greater, and the metacarpus is much arched or
contracted. This is seen in
conditions of exhaustion.

Two typical postures of
the hand still remain to be
described. The "hand in
fright" is a posture not often seen ; it is a modification
of the energetic hand, the
wrist and fingers being all
extended. It is well represented in the statue of Cain
(Fig. 13), and in several members of the Niobe Group at
Florence.

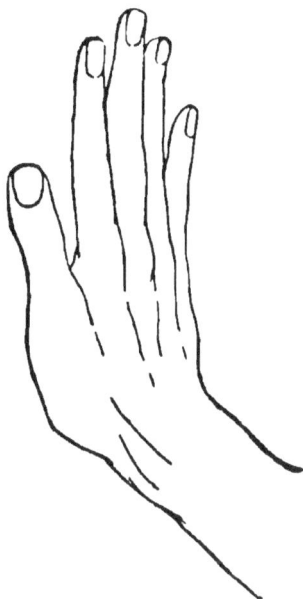

Fig. 11.—HAND IN FRIGHT.

When a child is convulsed
by epilepsy or brain disease, we usually see the hand

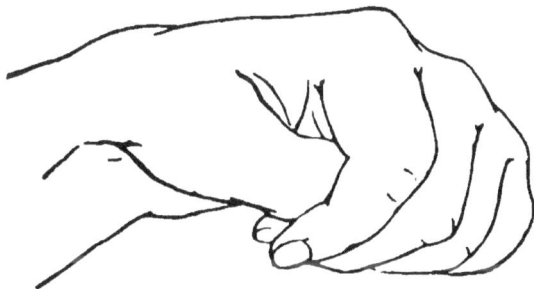

Fig. 12.—CONVULSIVE HAND.

clenched as a closed fist. The thumb is strongly flexed
on the palm of the hand, while the fingers are closed

over it, thus forming a closed fist, while the palm is
arched or contracted by bringing its sides together.
This position is never normal, but in a few cases
may occur as a sim-
ple matter of habit.
The convulsive hand
may be seen in a child
in passion, and it some-
times occurs during a
strong effort of self-
control; I have often
seen it in people when
about to have a tooth
drawn.

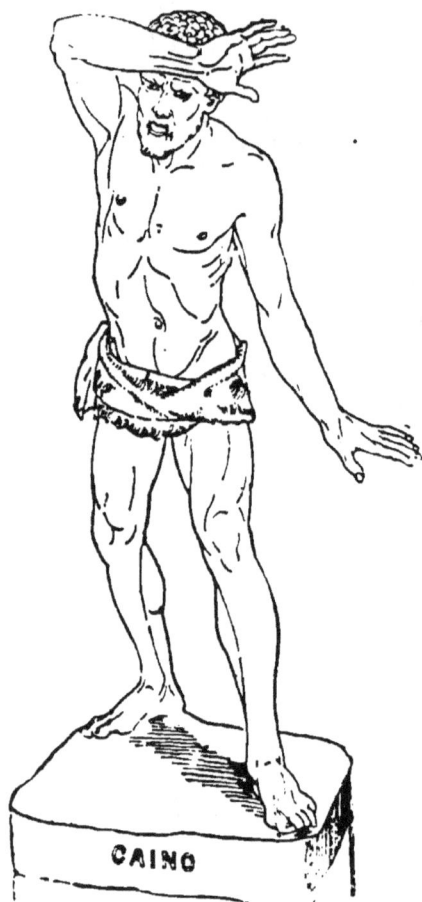

The eight types of
hand postures will
help you to describe
what you see, but va-
rious deviations from
these types will often
occur.

I ask your attention
to signs which are prob-
ably new to you, indi-
cating the brain-con-

CAINO

Fig. 13.

dition of children; that is, the study of postures or
attitudes of the body and limbs. Such signs will, I
think, be most useful to you, as they have been to me,

and, with a little practice, they are easily observed and described.

When the hand is held out, the posture or attitude seen is brought about by the last movements that occurred in the parts of the hand. Postures are, so to speak, stationary results of movement; the posture is the outcome of the balance of the muscles which produce it; and this is the outcome of the balance or ratio of action in the nerve-centres which stimulate the muscles to contract. Without going into theoretical matters, let me say that postures of the parts of the body are important signs of the brain-state at the time. The postures you see are most commonly due to, and are signs of, the condition of the nerve-system.

When I began to make the expression of conditions of the brain a definite study, I frequently looked at my patients, especially the children, after I had found out what their condition was, and I noted down any visible expression of their nerve-condition. My attention was soon attracted to the frequent occurrence of certain postures of the body indicative of conditions of the nerve-system. It is often more easy to describe postures than to describe movements; postures are conditions of quiescence; they can be watched during a space of time; they can be drawn, photographed, or represented by casts in plaster; movements are evanescent, like thoughts.

To study postures as signs of the mental brain-state
of the child, look at his parts and members when free
or disengaged. To observe the hand for this purpose,
it should not be engaged in holding a pen, but be free,
that all the fingers may move as the brain will move
them; that the brain-state, not the pen, may govern the
posture of the hand. The hand of a labourer[1] is seen
engaged in digging with his spade; his nerve muscular
energy is expended in holding and driving his spade.
It would, under such circumstances, require a very
strong nerve-current sent to those muscles to alter this
forcible brain-stimulus. Hence, the hand while engaged in digging, is not very impressionable and
expressive of the finer motor actions of the nerve-
mechanism. When the man puts aside his spade and
talks, especially if at rest, his hand gesticulates and
expresses his emotions. The hand may be said to be
free when it is held out at the word of command, when
hanging over the arm of a chair, or when it is moving
towards an object.

The face may usually be considered free to be acted
on only by the brain, except when eating. When a
strong cold wind blows on the face, it is too strongly
stimulated thereby, to be very impressionable to force
originating in the brain. The eyes are free when not
strongly stimulated by the sight of some object, or
bright light or colour.

[1] See "Physical Expression," p. 144.

In examining movement and balance, it is desirable that you should use the same word of command, the same stimulus to action, on all occasions. This action of the child is convenient, leaving the arms and hands free, and ready for your observation and description. It is desirable that the upper extremities, when thus under observation, should be free and unoccupied; they must not be engaged in doing anything. If I hold a lump of chalk in my hand, it is not free to express the condition of the brain. Clasping the hand on the chalk is partly a reflex act, following the pressure of the chalk; only in part is it due to the direct action of the brain upon the muscles of the limb.

If you see the hand of the child thus occupied, and you wish to observe it as a sign of brain-condition; either cause the hand to drop what it holds, or wait and watch for the favourable opportunity for your observations when the spontaneous action of the child shall set the hand free. The hand may be free when passing to reach an object, not so when it has seized it; it may be free when hanging over the arm of a chair, less so when resting on the table.

Looking at a body of children, say in the third or fourth standard, or grade, of a primary school, you will see, perhaps, five or ten per cent of them who do not present this perfect balance and typical posture. The appearance of certain deviations from this standard of the normal marks the child to me at once as probably

nervous, excitable, or exhausted. The observation of
certain groups of signs tells us something of the character or kind of child and his tendencies. It may be a
matter of interest and importance to those responsible
for children to look at them, study them, and observe
the presence of signs which indicate their present condition and probable tendencies in future development.

In observing movements as signs of brain-action, and
in describing them, it is most important to note the
parts moving. Movements may be seen principally in
the digits, more in these small parts than in larger
parts, such as the elbow and shoulder; they may be
seen principally in the muscles about the mouth, or in
certain other parts about the face. In any case, the
movement of a part corresponds to action in a certain
group of nerve-cells corresponding. Remember this
physiological fact, — it is the basis of much that is
important in the management of children. One series
of movements long continued means long continued
action of one portion of brain; change the action of the
child, and you thereby change the portion of brain
acting; thus you may help to avoid fatigue and
exhaustion.

I spoke just now of movements of small parts of
the body in contrast to movements of large parts. The
fine movements of small parts more directly indicate
brain-action; these should not only be carefully described by the observer, but also cultivated by the

teacher as in paper cutting, folding and similar occupations. I think the same kind of brain culture may be given by calisthenic exercises, which should be arranged not only to strengthen large muscles, but also to develop slight and independent movements of small parts of the body and the ready action of small portions of brain produced by imitation of your movements.

Looking at the arms of the child, observe the hands, wrists, elbows, shoulders on either side; look not only to the postures, but also to the movements. Postures and movements may be alike on either side, or they may be asymmetrical; you will find it not uncommon to have several signs of weakness on the same side of the body. When the two sides of the body do not move alike, it is commonly due to the diminished force or energy of brain, as seen in a tired child who leans on a table or chair.

Asymmetry of the postures of the body is usually accompanied by a slight tendency to lateral curvature of the spine. Postures of the spine are well worthy of study. As I have shown you, the spine is a column composed of many small bones, and is capable of being bent in various directions. Lateral curvature of the spine may be suspected if a child when at work constantly bends to one side, making one shoulder higher than the other. This may be due to weakness, and may be accompanied by finger twitching and weak hand postures unequal on the two sides. Stooping, or lateral bending of the spine, may be due to short sight or other eye defects, which should be looked for in such cases. When you notice a child bending over his work, get the test-type and examine him for short sight.

We have spoken of certain postures of the hand as being the opposite or antithesis of one another, and as representing opposite states of the nerve-system. We saw that the " nervous hand " was a posture the very opposite of that called the "energetic hand," and that these postures represent very different brain-states ; so with regard to the head, flexion or drooping indicates conditions the opposite of those expressed by extension or throwing backwards of the head.

The principles employed for the classification of movements are interesting not only as affording means of grouping many of the nerve-signs which you observe, but also in understanding the brain-action corresponding to what you see, and the brain-changes accompanying the emotions and other mental states, while they may help you in economising the child's nerve-force and preventing brain-fatigue.

We may class the movements we see as to their cause or according to what we think produced the action. Some movements are directly produced by and follow some stimulation from without. When the child is shown an object, his head, eyes, and hands move in that direction as he takes it ; sight regulates his movements, so when you call him he runs to you, stimulated by the sound of your voice which controls him. Typical examples of movements stimulated by impressions from outside the body, are seen in what the physiologist calls reflex actions. When the eyeball is touched, a stimulus is sent to the nerve-centre with the result that a nerve-current is quickly sent back from the nerve-cells to the muscles closing the eyes.

On the other hand, movements are often observed without· any known circumstances stimulating them; such are seen in the spontaneous movements of the infant and in the uncontrolled movements of the eyes and the finger twitches of fidgety children. Spontaneous movements are the chief characteristic of the condition called chorea.

We may, however, observe the characters of a movement itself apart from other circumstances. Looking at the face of a child, you may see the muscles in the forehead (frontals) working up and down making horizontal puckerings — a uniformly repeated, uncontrolled, senseless action; or again they may act momentarily, this may indicate a passing thought or feeling. Some children acquire " habits," such as holding the back of one hand to the forehead, or twisting one hand in a peculiar way again and again, or shrugging one shoulder, or turning the head, etc. Many foolish-looking habits in children consist in such uniformly repeated acts.

When action in several parts is observed, we have a combination and series of combinations of acts, making up a complex phenomenon; such series may be classified as follows, and the nerve-action corresponding may be indicated :

1. Uniformly repeated series of acts.

As when all the fingers are opened and closed together again and again. Here the same nerve-centres habitually act together.

2. Augmenting series of acts.

A spreading series of movements, corresponding to a spreading area of nerve-action may be seen in a spreading smile or facial expression, or a burst of laughter, and in the march of movement as from face to head and hand — in protrusion of the tongue on any stimulation ; in the head held on one side when any question is asked, and in the fidgety fingers of the examinee. Such spreading action is antithetical to good intellectual function.

This is much seen in the expression of emotion and in mental excitment and confusion : it corresponds to a wide area of brain in useless over-action and is exhausting.

3. A diminishing series of acts.

A diminishing series of acts with lessening of the area of motor cells in activity is seen in the child who is getting quieter after some excitement.

4. A series of acts adapted by circumstances.

In action adapted by circumstance, we have a high-class function commonly called coördinate action, and if the coördinating conditions were some time ante-cedent, the action is considered more strictly mental in character.

Brain-action thus fully controlled or coördinated is an economy of power, the force expended is adapted in its action by the environment and therefore probably in harmony with it.

A spreading area of brain in over-action is seen in stammering; here the spasm, accompanying and caus-ing the defect of speech, may be seen to commence in the muscles of the face about the angles of the mouth, in depression of the lower jaw, or in knitting of the eyebrows. Then the tongue is thrown into spasm, and, it may be, the muscles of respiration as well. The march of the spasm should be noticed; it usually recurs in the same order. On the first indication of visible spasm, which usually precedes the sound of the stam-mer, the child should be stopped in his effort to speak. Most of the children who stammer are boys.

A spreading area of movement may be healthy, as the resumption of spontaneity of action all over the body when children are let out to play; but such usually removes, for the time, the previous order or method of mental action. Laughter is another example of a spreading area of motor brain-action; it is apt to remove a line of thought. Could you induce the expression of joy and laughter in the boy in the first stage of anger,— say by imitation of you or of the other children,— much might be done to improve his mental status.

I think it must be evident from what has been said, that in many instances it is quite possible to observe the motor signs expressing mental states, and to deduce therefrom the modes of brain-action corresponding to such mental attitudes. I have not space to follow out this subject here.

If you succeed by your personal skill in improving the expression of the child in his movement and action, you have succeeded to some extent, at least, in improving his brain, removing its disorderliness, increasing thereby mental and moral aptitude. Training, adapted to such purpose, differs from many of the modes of physical training commonly employed in schools. To improve the action of the child's brain by physical exercises, he should be trained rather by his sight in imitation of the teacher's movements, than by drill conducted by the word of command or by music. Marching and exercises with dumb-bells, poles, or clubs, as well as with the closed fists, are very useful means of increasing muscular power and improving the chest. To coördinate or regulate the brain by physical training, " free exercises " are needed. There should be nothing in the hands as they move.

CHAPTER VI

In Chapter IV., I referred to the parts of the child you should look at, and described what to look for among normal signs; giving a schedule to assist your description. While looking at each part and the action and movement, faulty signs may be seen; these should be described verbally on that schedule, or they may be recorded conveniently on the subjoined form of card.

In the card, the main classes of defect are printed, viz. : A. Development Defects. B. Nerve-signs. C. Nutrition (defective). D. Dull.

As points among development defects we have (1) Cranium or head, and the sub-classes of type of defect of head. (11) External ear. (12) Epicanthis. (13) Palate, and its sub-classes of type of defect.

As points among nerve-signs we have (43) General balance; action in the face (44–48); also, movements of the eyes; balance of the head and the hands, etc.

The more common faults in body or in brain action are those briefly indicated on the card with a reference number, referring to detailed description of the sign, given below.

The card is intended for use in describing a child presenting any bodily or brain faults seen; it is convenient for reference — the points seen to be faulty being indicated quickly by passing the pen through the names of the defects present. At the right-hand lower corner of the card is a formulated epitome ABCD EFG on which the main classes of defect present in the child may be recorded by passing the pen through the symbols corresponding.

Description of these faults or defects will now be given (p. 99).

Points for Observation describing Faults or Defect in Body or Brain Status.

The principal signs of defect are here described, with remarks as to their significance. The numbers refer to the card.

A. **Defects in Development.** — The term includes any point of defect in the form, proportion, or size of the body and its parts, or the absence of any part.

(*a* 1) **Cranium Defective** includes any defect in size, form, proportion of the head. At seven years the head should measure 20 inches in circumference. Of all defects in development those of the cranium or head appear to be the most important, having the closest relation with other kinds of defect. The size and the probable volume of the brain is a point of first-class

School............... Card No...........

St¹................ .... Reg. No............ BOYS.

Age .... Spl. Rep¹.............

A	DEVELOPMENT DEFECTS		47	O. oculi lax	
a	1	CRANIUM	48	Eye-movements	
	2	Large	49	Head-balance	
	3	Small	50	Hand weak	
	4	Bossed	51	Hand nervous	
	5	Forehead	52	Finger twitches	
	6	Frontal ridge	53	Lordosis	
			h 54	OTHER NERVE-SIGNS	
b	11	EXTERNAL EAR			
c	12	EPICANTHIS	**C**	NUTRITION	
d	13	PALATE	**D**	DULL	
	14	Narrow	**E**	EYE-CASES	
	15	V-shaped	64	Squint	
	16	Arched	65	Glasses plus	
	17	Cleft	66	Glasses minus	
	18	Other types	67	Myopia, no glasses	
e	19	NASAL BONES	68	Cornea disease	
f	20	GROWTH SMALL	69	Eye, lost accident	
g	21	OTHER DEVELMT. DFTS.	70	Eye, lost disease	
B	NERVE-SIGNS		**F**	RICKETS	
	43	General balance	**G**	EXCEPTIONAL CHILDREN	
	44	Expression	i 82	CRIPPLES	
	45	Frontals overact			
	46	Corrugation		A B C D E F G	

importance, and the size of the head is, in children, a fair indication of the size of the brain.

It also appears that defects in the form of the head are often accompanied with weakness or lessened brain-power. Defects of the cranium are divided into sub-classes.

(*a* 2) **Cranium Large.** — A head of 22 inches circumference or over is large in a school child; allowance must be made for age. Large heads are sometimes accompanied by the signs of rickets.

(*a* 3) **Cranium Small.** — The point of size of head is recorded as apart from the size of the child for its age. The volume is estimated in relation to the normal for age. This is determined by inspection, by the open hand placed upon the head, and by the measuring tape. A head with a circumference over 20 inches at any school age is not registered as small; usually the small heads are 18 to $19\frac{1}{2}$ inches circumference. Small head is noted independent of stature.

In this group, contrary to the usual rule, the defect is more common among girls. If there be no other defect, mental faculty may be average, but the child usually remains thin and delicate; such children may, in after life undertake good work and do it, but are more liable than others to exhaustion, headaches, and breakdown of the nerve-system. At school these children are often delicate and irregular in attendance for ailments.

(*a* 4) **Cranium Bossed.** — There may be bosses, protuberances, or outgrowths of bone on the two halves of the forehead or elsewhere. These are usually alike on the two sides, but not always. These bosses are probably largely due to rickets; were all possible means adopted for the prevention of rickets, we should probably have fewer children with cranial abnormalities and dull brains.

(*a* 5) **Forehead Defective.** — The forehead may be narrow, shallow in vertical measurement, or small in all dimensions; it may bulge forward and overhang. All defects of the forehead, except "bosses" and "frontal ridge" (*a* 4, *a* 6) are here included.

(*a* 6) **Frontal Ridge.**— There may be a bony ridge projecting vertically under the skin down the middle of the forehead. This sign is not very important, unless accompanied by a narrow and shallow forehead.

All these forms of defect of cranium are much more common among boys than girls, except the small head, which occurs mostly among girls in towns. Other less frequent types of defect of cranium are omitted as being of only medical importance.

(*b* 11) **External Ear** may be defective in its parts, size, and form. The ear may be outstanding and large, with great convexity behind, and the pleat of the ear (antehelix) may be absent as well as the whole or part of the curled rim of the ear; the skin over the ear may be coarse, red, and liable to chilblains in the winter. The ears may not be both alike; the lobe of the ear may be adherent to the face in place of drooping. Such defects have no necessary connection with dull hearing. Defective ears are much more frequently seen in boys than in girls.

(c 12) **Eyelids with Epicanthis.** — The epicanthis is a fold of skin continuous with the lower fold of the upper eyelid (not a fold of mucous membrane) placed across the inner angle of the opening of the eyelids; it may be asymmetrical.

(d 13) **Defective Condition of Palate.** — Defect of the palate, though less frequent than that of the cranium, stands next to it, as being of the greatest importance.

The principal defects of palate are in its proportions as seen in the horizontal or vertical plane. Without being otherwise altered the palate may be contracted laterally or narrow. The V-shaped palate is pointed more or less sharply at its anterior extremity, the lines of the upper jaw being nearly straight, meeting anteriorly at an acute angle. The high-arched or vaulted palate deviates from the normal in the vertical plane.

(d 14) **Palate Narrow.** — Without being otherwise altered, the palate may be contracted laterally in the space between the teeth.

(d 15) **V-shaped Palate.** — Pointed more or less sharply at its anterior extremity, the lines of the upper jaw being nearly straight lines, meeting at their extremities at an acute angle.

(*d* 16) **Palate Arched** or Vaulted, thus deviating from the normal in the vertical plane with a high roof.

(*d* 17) **Palate Cleft.** — A deformity which may affect the hard and the soft palate.

(*e* 19) **Nasal Bones** wide, sunken, or indented. The bony bridge of the nose may be thus ill-shapen and depressed. It must be remembered that in the infant the bony part of the nose projects but little and does not grow out prominently, till three or four years old. When the deformity exists, it may be accompanied by obstruction in the throat or nose, and deafness.

(20) **Growth Small.** — Children short and small in build for their age or dwarfed. The stature of the child should be observed as apart from the size of the head : the head may be small, and the child tall, or *vice versa*. See Table II. as to normal height.

The relations of this condition appear to indicate that small grown children are at a disadvantage. Many of the children with small heads are small in growth also, but the number of children with small heads is much larger than the number with small growth. This is an example where normal proportion in the body is not to the child's advantage ; the small child is probably better fitted for after life, when his head is full sized.

Some of these small grown children are badly grown as the result of rickets.

(21) **Other Development Defects** includes points not printed on the card; the more important of them are described below.

(26) **Face Small.** — The face as a whole may be small, including the upper and lower jaws, and that independent of the size of the upper part of. the head, which contains the brain.

(27) **Features Coarse, Heavy, Flat.** — The features may be large and ill-proportioned. The separate features may not be individually malformed, but disproportionate one to another or to the size of the face: thus the nose may be small; the face large, round, flat, the features rising from the plane of the face; the lips may be thick and protuberant.

(28) **Forehead Hairy.** — The forehead may be covered with fine downy hair; the hairy scalp may join the outer extremities of the eyebrows.

(30) **Hands Blue and Cold.** — This may be seen in some children, even in the summer; it is commonly associated with defectiveness.

(34) **Mouth Small.** — The mouth as seen when at rest, may be too small; this is sometimes accompanied by obstruction of nose or throat with deafness.

(39) **Eye Openings Defective** in size or form. The eyelids may be small, as well as the openings between them, both in their vertical and transverse measurements. In some cases the opening is not symmetrical, being wider on the inner than on its outer half.

The transverse axis may slope outwards and upwards, or outwards and downwards, instead of being horizontal.

B. **Abnormal Nerve-signs** as seen in balance and action in face, eye-movements, postures of the head and hands, and in response, etc.

(43) **General Balance Irregular.** — Not erect and straight, but slouching and listless. The shoulders not held at equal height, back bent or twisted over to one side, the feet not each planted similarly on the floor. When the hands are held out, they may be at a different level; more often the left is held lower than the right, and the left hand more nearly approaches the weak posture.

The balance of the body is thus not equal on the two sides.

(44) **Expression of Face Defective.** — Want of changefulness, vacancy, fixed expression.

We may describe the visible muscular action seen in a face, and still there may be an expression in it which entirely baffles description. Further, a face may be balanced or moved abnormally by the action of certain muscles, and yet it may carry upon it a good expression. We may describe action in the frontal muscles, the corrugators, the orbicularis oculi etc., and, over and above this, we have the general expression of the face superadded. Certain terms are useful in describing expression; there may be a fixed expression, want of variation, *i.e.* one fixed uniform action or balance of muscular tone; or we may have to use more general terms such as "defective," "bad." There may be no expression, *i.e.* none other than that indicated by form or modelling of the features.

(45) **Frontal Muscles over-acting.** — There is a pair of muscles in the forehead, placed vertically under the skin and attached at the eyebrows; by their action they raise the eyebrows, and produce horizontal creases in the forehead, which may be shallow or deep, making transverse puckers; in other cases the action is fine, producing minute creases, and what may be called a dull forehead. If this frequently occurs, it is a bad sign in children and is most common in those of unoccupied mind and untrained mental action.

This muscular over-action does not necessarily erase expression. Such over-action may be seen in children from earliest infancy upwards; the condition may be temporary, and, having lasted a sufficient number of years to produce permanent creases in the forehead, it may pass away. These muscles are often more quiet when the child is at work or being talked to, than when let out to play; the mental attitude, termed quiet attention, is that under which the frontal area is the most quiet.

This sign is far more frequent in boys than in girls.

(46) **Corrugation.** — Knitting the eyebrows; drawing the eyebrows together. There is a pair of muscles

in the forehead, placed horizontally between the eyebrows which draws them together, thus producing
vertical creases which may be deep or shallow, producing vertical puckerings on the forehead above the
nose, or only a fine wrinkling of the skin, which
contributes to a dull appearance of the forehead.
Corrugation (knitting eyebrows) may coexist with over-
action of the frontal muscles (frowning), producing
a puzzled expression, or, if deep, a "scowl," as in
ill-temper.

This sign seems more closely associated than any
other single sign with some forms of mental stress,
and may be seen in children suffering from the effects
of fright, illusions, etc.; it may form parts of a fixed
immobile expression.

This sign is more common in boys than girls.

(47) **Orbicularis Oculi relaxed.** — Fulness under the
eyes. There is a thin muscle (the orbicularis oculi) which
encircles the eyelids, and being attached to the skin gives
tone to the lower lid, so that its convexity is seen. In
a strong and well-toned face the lower lid appears clean-
cut and well moulded, the rotundity of the eyeball and
convexity of the lower lid are shown in sharp definition of outline, due to good tone in this muscle; in
smiling and laughter this muscle causes puckering of
the lower lid. When this muscle is relaxed and toneless, the skin of the under lid bulges forward and is
baggy, causing fulness under the eyes. This condition

is removed temporarily on making the child smile or laugh. The fulness under the eyes is indicative of fatigue, exhaustion, or low brain power in children: it frequently accompanies recurring headaches.

(48) **Eye-movements Defective.** — When an object is moved at a distance two feet in front of the face, the eyes should move in following it. In some children the head always turns towards the object while the eyes are kept still in their orbits. In other cases fixation of the eyes is bad, or there are restless uncontrolled movements of the eyes.

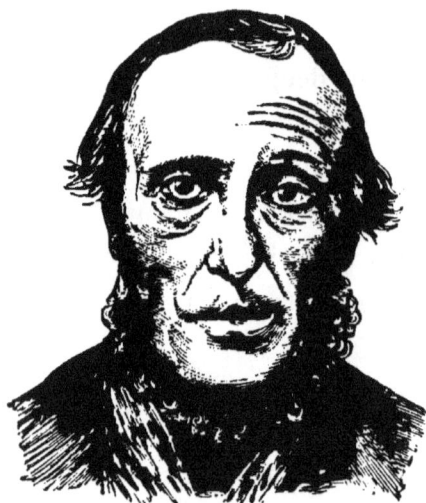

Fig. 14. — COMPLETE PARALYSIS OF THE RIGHT SIDE OF THE FACE. — The muscles of the face act only on the left side. In the forehead the frontal muscles produce horizontal furrows; the muscles about the mouth draw the left angle upwards; the eyelids are more widely separated on the right side.

Movements of the eyes not controlled as to their number and direction by obvious circumstances, must be looked upon as signs of nervousness. Irregular movements of the eyes are common in children, and are very indicative of the brain condition: they may be looked upon as analogous to spontaneous twitchings of the fingers.

In these wandering, irregular movements of the eyes
we find an illustration of a common law that excessive movement is often an indication of weakness not
of strength: the same thing is seen in the twitching
movements of nervous
children.

(49) **Head-balance.**—
The head should be
held erect; it may be
inclined to one side or
drooped forward. Ir-
regular balance of the
head is more common
in girls than in boys.

(50) **Hand-balance
Weak.**—In this type of
balance the hand when
held out is slightly
drooped or flexed at the
wrist, the palm slightly
contracted or arched
laterally, and the fin-
gers moderately flexed.

Fig. 15.— PARALYSIS OF RIGHT SIDE OF
FACE FROM BRAIN DISEASE. — The
face is not symmetrical, and the muscles on the right side about the mouth
act weakly. The line from the nose to
the mouth on this side is almost lost:
this is well seen on comparing the two
sides. Muscular action in the upper
and middle parts of the face is unequal
on each side.

The type may be varied: with less degrees of weakness the hand is as in the normal with the thumb
drooped only; in exhaustion or great feebleness the
palm is more contracted or adducted, and the degree
of flexion is greater.

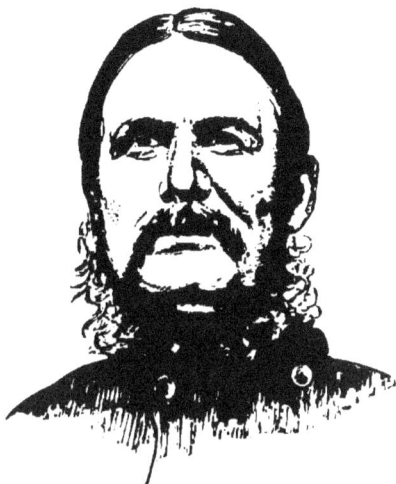

A bad type is seen when children holding out their hands droop both thumbs and bring them together in the median plane.

(51) **Hand-balance Nervous.** — In this posture the wrist is slightly drooped or flexed, the palm of the hand slightly contracted laterally, the thumb extended backwards, and the fingers at the knuckles are bent backwards (see Fig. 6).

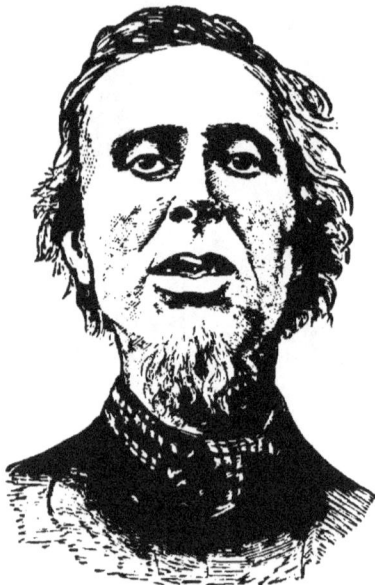

The various elements in this posture may vary in degree; the most essential element appears to be the extension backwards of the fingers at the knuckle joint, and this may affect the various fingers differently.

It is common with children with slight chorea, those the subjects of night-terrors and tooth-grinding, also accompanying recurrent headaches. It has been represented by artists in antique bronzes and drawings on vases, as well as in modern works, especially in female figures.

Fig 16. — PARALYSIS OF LEFT SIDE OF FACE FROM BRAIN DISEASE. — Similar differences are seen about the mouth. The eyelids are a little wider open on the left side.

(52) **Finger Twitches.** — When the hands are held

out for inspection, there may be twitching movements in the fingers. These may be up and down (flexion

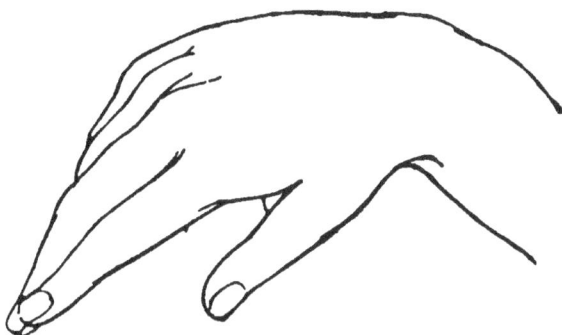

Fig. 17. — FEEBLE HAND.

and extension) or lateral; the latter are produced by the small muscles placed in the hand which pull the fingers sideways.

(53) **Lordosis.** — When the hands are held forward, an alteration in the balance of the spine may appear, with an arching forward in the lower part of the back, while the upper part of the spine between the shoulders is thrown back. This arching forward of the lumbar spine is due to weakness of action among the spinal muscles. When a child holds out his hands, the centre of gravity of the body is moved forward; in a strong child this is not followed by marked change of posture in the spine, but in a weak child lordosis may follow often with temporary lateral curvature and unequal balance of the shoulders while the head and neck are thrown back.

(54) **Other Abnormal Nerve-signs** include signs not printed on the card as being less frequent in occurrence than those given earlier, but not of less importance.

(55) **Deaf.** — Children deaf or partially so.   For tests of hearing see Chapter II.

(56) **Grinning or Over-smiling.** — In the lower part of the face you may see grinning or over-smiling about the angles of the mouth, temporarily widening the opening; the lines on the face may be slight or deep. Over-smiling or grinning is usually symmetrical, but may be unequal on the two sides of the face.

With low-class brain-conditions it is sometimes seen as almost the only facial movement occurring upon any stimulus as a uniform movement, almost as frequent as over-action of the frontal muscles.

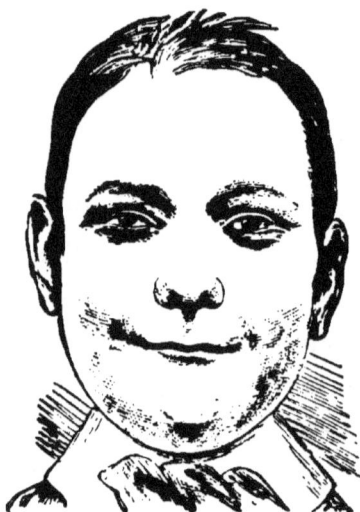

Fig. 18. — IMBECILE. — Head well shapen and of fair size; he often smiled, thus moving parts around the eyes and mouth.

If habitual, grinning and in particular the finer forms of over-smiling, often leave permanent naso-labial creases marked upon the skin, these may remain after the habit has been lost.   If the skin be thin, a duplicate or triplicate naso-labial crease may be formed:

this is more common in neurotic than in imbecile subjects.

(58) **Over-mobile.** — Constant spontaneous movements. Among children in the infant school and in some over seven years of age, spontaneous movement is the normal and a natural sign of healthy brain-activity ; it is most common in the eyes and the fingers. See spontaneous movements in infants, Chapter III. When spontaneous movements cannot be controlled, even temporarily, but are increased (extra-movements) when the child is spoken to, the condition passes on to that of chorea, which is more common in girls than boys. See chorea, Chapter XII.

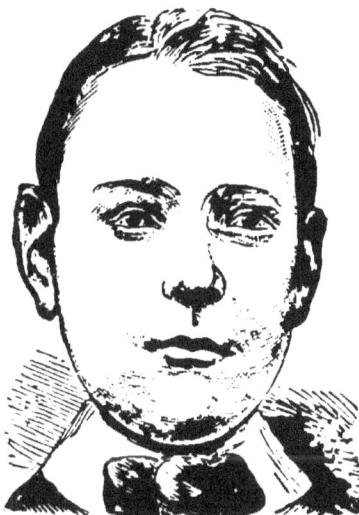

Fig. 19. — IMBECILE. — The same case quiescent ; face wanting expression.

(59) **Response in Action Defective.** — Dealing with groups of children by a uniform method of examination as described, it becomes easy to note the response to the word of command as seen in the action following. Response in action may be accurate or uncertain, there may be delay between hearing the command and the response ; some children look at the others before responding in their movements ; they

I

seem more easily controlled through the eye than the ear.

The response should be quick and accurate; the standard to be expected is soon learnt by a little experience. The action may be long continued, the hands of the child being held out long after the others have dropped them. There may be want of impressionability to the stimulus of the command, which may have to be repeated before the action follows; response in imitation by sight may be, and often is, much better than that following the word of command. There are some children in whom the sound of a command may be followed by a number of irregular movements, whereas an indication through the eye, by a gesture of command on the part of the inspector, is quickly followed by accurate and good response.

(60) **Speech Defective.** — Defective conditions of palate are consistent with good speech; an impediment is not usually the mechanical effect of the form of palate. It does, however, often happen that with defect of speech we find an arched or a narrow palate with co-existent brain-feebleness.

Utterance may be thick and indistinct owing to conditions of the throat and nose : observe if the child be a mouth-breather, usually keeping the lips parted for breathing and unable to keep them closed with comfort. These mouth-breathing children with thick speech often have large tonsils and conditions of the throat leading to deafness, which require medical treatment. The speech of children is very important; it may be almost absent, or accompanied by stammering or impediment. On putting a question it may be long before the reply comes, the question may be repeated without further reply; speaking to the child may be followed by a large number of irregular movements and asymmetrical postures, — awkward action, — but not by a verbal reply.

The voice may vary greatly in tone, falling to an almost inaudible whisper, in place of being well sustained; or too monotonous as a result of want of training, while the words are badly spaced as he speaks.

Speech is the most important mode of mental expression; it is a faculty that needs cultivation in all children. Indistinctness of speech is very common, and defects of speech are frequently met with, both in children generally healthy and well made, and in others of defective constitution.

Stammering is a defect in articulating certain sounds, and is due to a defect in the nerve-system, often associated with other faulty conditions of brain; it is much more commonly met with in boys than girls, and to some extent may be acquired through imitation among children, predisposed by their inheritance. Stammering presents visible muscular spasm in the face and other parts, usually commencing and spreading in a uniform order in the same boy, but varying in different cases. The attack consists, essentially, in a temporary spasm or rigidity of certain muscles which prevents them from being properly controlled by the brain. When the boy stammers on commencing to speak, he almost immediately stops on uttering certain sounds, because the muscles used in articulation become rigid; the range of the spasm and the groups of muscles affected may vary in different cases. In the attack the mouth may quiver, often more on one side; the jaw is then depressed, and as the mouth is opened, the tongue may be seen in tremor with the tip near the front teeth, while the trembling of the tongue-muscles may be felt by the finger placed under the chin. Other muscles in the face may be affected: the eyebrows are often knit (corrugation), and an expression of distress may be seen. These recurrent spasms in the face may leave lines in the skin, marking the boy as a stammerer.

The attempt to remove stammering by training must be long and patiently continued; the employment of general physical exercises quietly conducted, and training in full breathing may be useful. Every prolonged attack of stammering tends to its recurrence. A most important point is to lessen the duration and severity of each attack, and to arrest the spasm, when it commences; that is to say, let the boy stop speaking at the moment, and try again presently. The teacher should then learn to observe the usual sign of commencing spasm and stop speaking at once. These children may sing without difficulty.

Case 15. A boy who stammers: muscular spasm commences in the forehead.

A school-boy eleven years of age was brought to me, because he had been liable to stammer for the last four years, this trouble having been increased the last three weeks, coincident with disturbed digestion. On asking him a simple question he stammered in his reply. Looking at his face, the following conditions were seen. When about to stammer, the muscles in the forehead produced both horizontal and vertical furrows; in the lower part of the face the mouth was widened on either side, together with elevation of the upper lip opposite the canine tooth; this was more marked on the right than the left side.

Case 16. Stammerer; muscular spasm commences about the mouth, an intelligent boy — rickets.

A boy twelve years of age, intelligent, but stammers badly. This does not interfere with singing, and he has joined a choir. He is tall, rather thin, weight 5½ stones (77 lbs.). The head and chest show signs of rickets in infancy, probably resulting from the fact that he was fed on biscuits as a baby. His general balance of body is faulty, and his hands are not held out straight; physical training may improve his action.

On beginning to speak, spasm in the face commences at the right angle of the mouth, and saliva dribbles from it; the spasm then spreads and the forehead becomes puckered; the mouth opens and the tongue is seen quivering against the teeth, while his colour heightens during the attack. He was placed at a small school near the sea and improved in health with some improvement of speech.

CHAPTER VII

EXAMINATION OF MENTAL ABILITY AND THE FAULTS THAT MAY BE OBSERVED

WHEN examining a child's mental ability in school, you will naturally speak to him and let him talk to you as well as read and write, if he is old enough. The proper use of speech is a most important indication of the mental processes; but we shall see that other tests not involving speech, reading or the use of figures, are also of great interest.

Let the child stand, and holding his book in a good light read a passage to you. Notice how the book is held and whether it is kept 18 inches or so from his face: if he shows difficulty or is timid, it may be well that you should read the passage to him first or read it with him; or better take a passage you know, and recite it, watching his face and his eyes.

Talk to the child and let him talk to you of his home, his amusements, games, pet animals, pocket-money, and the stories he reads; you can observe the while the child's expression and speech, his control by hearing and accuracy in seeing. In his talk you may notice how far he can express himself in words and speak connectedly: in his answers to questions you observe whether his processes of thinking are orderly and natural. A young child tends to repetition of the words of the question, especially if he sees the face of the speaker; this is by no means a point of defect at an early age, and proves that the child heard the question; but in some children, old enough to do better, the question is simply repeated or imitated without any attempt at reply. Repetition of the question shows imitation and delayed mental action in place of a prompt mental process; if the subsequent answer is correct, the delay does not very much matter, but sometimes the delay is so long, that the impress of the question (auditory) on the brain fades and no true thinking results. If this delay in response is accompanied by extra-movements and fidgetiness, a mental fault (probably mental confusion) is indicated.

The child's vocabulary may be very limited, comparatively few words having been acquired, — perhaps 200; this is sometimes owing to the child having been allowed to point to things wanted instead of asking for them, just as he may grow up lazy and backward by having all his wants anticipated for him by others. To increase the number of words habitually used and available for language, correctly employed, is an important part of mental

training and improves brain-power and the capacity
for thinking : perhaps vocabulary is best extended by
talking to and with the child — we must not wait for
him to get his words from books. Speech and articulation need training in all children ; speech may be
too monotonous, not modulated in tone and indistinct;
the spacing of words in speaking and reading may
be badly arranged. Good speaking is very indicative
of good mental aptitude well trained ; to impart good
faculty in speech gives an important form of mental
refinement.

A talk with the child may be planned to show
many mental characteristics. Social and moral sense
should be looked for in the child, and knowledge
how to act correctly in social life, as well as how
to avail himself of common social methods under
varying circumstances. Can the child write a letter?
Ask him what he must get before he can write the
letter, how he buys the stamps, how the letter gets
to the person to whom it is addressed; ask him how
he would get there himself and what money would
be wanted. The child's ideas as to how he would
protect himself from danger, how he would try to
help another child, and what he would do with a
dog, may show much.

Memory may be tested by asking the home address, the day of the week and the month, and past
common events probably within the child's experience

—ask him where he puts his books and keeps other things, when done with, and how he finds them again, whether he looks for them or asks some one else to do so. The child that uses his eyes badly is apt to have a bad memory : this form of mental association of ideas (brain-centres in co-action) that gives memory is largely produced by accurate seeing (impress of brain through the eye).

Test the pupil in his knowledge of the use of numbers and in arithmetic, both on paper and by simple calculations worked in his head. Is he more accurate when he looks at figures on the slate and uses his eyes or when he does mental arithmetic without the help of his eyes? again in the latter attempt does he count on his fingers? Some children of low mental ability have a great faculty for remembering figures, and sometimes in making certain calculations.

Some power of reasoning may be tested by describing common objects, pointing out in what particulars they can be compared. Show a pin and a pencil. Are they alike? If the pupil tells you that the pin is small and the pencil larger, and that each is much longer than it is wide, that indicates a mental comparison and a judgment.

Imitation is faculty involving brain-action which is principally effected through sight : the objects imitated by the child in school are the teacher's actions, expressions, gestures, movements, and those of the other pupils. Test the child's brain-power in imitation of your action. Let the child stand and look at you, telling him to do as you do. When you hold out your right hand, the child holds out his left, which is opposite to your right; the side of movement is thus reversed throughout the exercise, unless he has otherwise been trained; this is the instinctive mode of response. Make your movements with care and accuracy, noting what you do; see that the child looks at your hand, not at your face or eyes, and observe if his movements in imitation are exactly the same as yours, in the parts he moves, in the time and quickness of movement, and in the degree or quantity of movement.

Let me suggest a few finger exercises for your use in thus testing the children, and for convenience I will name the fingers thus: A, the thumb; B, the index finger; C, the middle finger; D, the ring finger; E, the little finger.

Make the following order of movements slowly and separately one after the other:

A, bend thumb; A and B; A, B, and C; B, C, D, E; E only.

B, index finger, moved from side to side without bending it up or down.

C, middle finger moved in the same manner.

Thus vary your movements while the pupil follows you, as a well-trained child will do. In this and in many other ways you may test with accuracy the power of imitation and control of movements by sight of your action.

After talking to the child and observing his movements in imitation, you will probably find, as is usually the case, some analogy between the two modes of brain-action, movement and thinking. The child who is slow in all his actions and in speech is apt to be slow in his mental processes. He may be slow in movement, holding out his hands long after the command, while he looks to see what others do before he does the same, and will keep his hands out after the others have dropped theirs : class-practice is useful to quicken such children. He also takes a long time to make a simple calculation in his head or to work with figures on paper; he is slow in thinking out the answer to a simple question and in expressing in words what he really knows, the words do not form quickly in his brain, as in other children; at the same time a brightening expression in the face may suggest that a mental process is going on there : though long in answering he may at length do so correctly.

A child's mental process may be too slow and limited, though fairly accurate. The interval between speaking to him and the reply may be too long. Then try not only to quicken his mental processes, but also to quicken the interaction of the eye, the ear, and the hand, as by games, and especially competitive games with a ball where the action must be quick or failure follows.

A child may not be really slow in the processes of thinking, but an impression having been made on the brain, its expression in action or in words may occur at a later time. The child may see or hear something and act upon it or talk about it another time; there may be delayed expression of a mental impression.

Case 17. A child, four years old, looked quietly at his mother putting a letter into a pillar-box; she could not at the time see the impression made upon the child's brain, but thought some impression had been produced, because his head and eyes turned towards the pillar-box: she knew next day that an impression had been received, when the child seeing a letter on the table took it and posted it behind the door — an action he had not been known to do previously.

In older children expression of thought may be long delayed; the pupil begins to answer some former question, as to which some half-unconscious mental process has been going on. A question may be asked in class and not answered; later on some reply to that question is given unconsciously, when another question is put. "How does a plant get the water for its leaves?" No answer. "What is the shape of this leaf?" *Ans.* "Oval, with a midrib, and the water comes to the pulp of the leaf along that, and the root draws the water from the ground." The pupil knew about it all the time; the association of ideas suggested by the second question completed the correct processes of thinking.

The term Introspection is used to imply the habit in a child of thinking about his own thoughts — his own thoughts being the subject of his contemplation, rather than the thoughts implanted at school, or his games and the common objects of interest to children. Such children will ask you how a stone was made, or put to you a problem of ethics, which may puzzle you, and is a useless point for the child to think about. This habit in a child is, sometimes, very exhausting to the brain-power, particularly when practised in a half-dormant state. Serious thinking about the mental state, goodness and what ought to be, should, I think, be undertaken only when the mental faculties are at their brightest and under the guidance of a trained mind, so that, under friendly advice, some immediate good action may follow. Introspection is found as a habit among children of the nervous class, and is largely due to want of proper guidance and mental control. If it recurs often, it may be well to give the child some concrete thought which he may be taught to recall, when his thoughts thus wander, as often they do on trying to fall asleep. Let him call up in imagination some pleasant landscape scene, a game, or the sight of his mother, or other subject not bad to dream on. Muscular activity during the day and a school-life among other children may remove such habits of thinking, and useless waste of strength. This spontaneous thinking in a child, not in accordance with his environment, seems to me to be very analogous to the spontaneous movements of infancy; it effects nothing, but is a sign of mental action, which needs to be coördinated and directed.

Children of the kind here referred to are sometimes said to be precocious and clever; I suspect that these self-contained thoughts do not do much good.

Mental ability in knowledge, calculation, memory, and in reasoning power may be tested by questions asked of the pupil; failure to pass such tests may show ignorance or the absence of previous training, or it may be want of mental faculty. Again, mental tests by question and answer are not well adapted to prove mental ability or its absence in very young children. We then have to look for other points by which to estimate brain-power for mental processes, especially applicable to children dull or backward, and neglected, or difficult in receiving instruction.

In testing the brain-faculty we need not rely solely on questions and answers, whether oral or written. A child, untrained in school work, may appreciate number, weight, size, colour, form, though he has not the ready use of words for describing what he understands: we may find that he has brain-faculty in imitation, in power of exercising choice, making comparison and in judgment.

Let the child count some money as it lies on the table, first as to the number of pieces, then sort the coins as to their metal, and as to value; he may show mental capacity in the process. To be more accurate in such examination, let the pupil count the coins with his own hands, one by one, on to the pile, *i.e.* count his hand-movements; let him count them again, as you place them one by one in a pile, *i.e.* count your hand-movements by moving his eyes. Again let him count the coins as they lie on the table, without touching them, by his eye-movements alone. Note by which method he proceeds best. Can he name or distinguish coins without seeing them when placed in his open hands, on the palm or on his fingers; feeling their weight and comparing them (muscular sense), or must he close his fingers on them and appreciate them by his finger-movements (sense of movements of small parts)?

Test his knowledge of various weights; use $\frac{1}{4}$, $\frac{1}{2}$, 1 oz. weights. It is convenient to use iron weights where the size is proportional to the weight, and also pill-boxes all of the same size and appearance, the weights being made up by plaster inside. Let the child weigh each in his hands, with the fingers open, and again closing his fingers over the object and feeling its size; he may thus form a judgment and comparison of weight. He may not only form a judgment as to the proportion of weights, but also name a single weight given to him: this is an act of memory and proper use of names.

You may also test the sense of temperature by warming a coin in hot water and see if he appreciates its warmth.

Case 18. A dumb boy acquired experience and reasoning as to temperature.

I detected acquired experience and some reasoning power in a small boy almost without speech thus: I touched his hand with a piece of metal, and he looked at me, then letting him see me heat the metal in some steaming hot water, he very properly declined to let me touch him again with that piece of metal; but he took a ball from me readily and played with it. This boy was capable of gaining experience and acting on it in self-defence.

Case 19. A very dull boy, short-sighted, and deaf, can compare weights.

A boy, eight years of age, has always been delicate and backward; he attends a Kindergarten and has begun reading words of two or three letters, paper-folding, colouring; he knows copper coins from one another and is fond of singing. He is timid, but social and not troublesome. His speech is thick and nasal so as to be hardly intelligible, but he tries to speak; the mouth is small, while the lips are thick and never quite closed. He is small and short for his age; weight 3 st. 4 lb. (46 lb.); height 3 ft. 8 in. His

K

head is small, only 18½ inches circumference, and the palate is narrow. Facial expression is wanting, with fulness under his eyes and horizontal frowning; the hands balance in the "nervous posture"; he can put pins in a cushion one by one, but is slow and clumsy. Looking at my watch, he places his face horizontal, holding the watch six inches from his eyes. The boy is small-brained, delicate, short-sighted, and has obstruction in his throat interfering with breathing and hearing. He has faculty in judgment, for he compared weights accurately; and told me himself that the iron weight was cold.

As a further test of accuracy in movement let the child try to touch his nose with his eyes shut, then other parts of his face, eye, and ear, as you name them; again with his left hand held out and the fingers spread, let him shut his eyes and with the index finger of his right hand touch the fingers on his left hand, one after another, naming them if he can.

Accuracy in telling the time by a clock or by your watch is a useful test; you may detect short sight in the child, who can see the clock at two feet, but cannot read the watch at ten inches.

In examining any child, his handwriting is worth preserving; let him write his name and address with the date.

Teachers who deal with mental state mainly, generally know more of the mental than of the physical and general brain-state of their pupils; in school inspection we find it more easy to detect physical and general brain-states. A child may have grave mental defects and may yet present no obvious defects that the eye of the observer can detect. Questioning and somewhat prolonged examination is needed to detect mental defects, when no obvious signs are observable. The physical observer may be sure of the signs he observes, but to see no defects does not prove that the child is normal.

Looking back at the mental examination of the pupil, let us see what principles are involved in the tests applied. This we may do by tracing motor action, point by point, corresponding to the expression of mental acts or status, and infer the kind of brain-action that takes place corresponding to each. Thus: The child is inaccurate in reading and slips a line, as he fails to carry his eye correctly from the end of one line to the beginning of the next; this may be due to untrained eye-movements, not to mental dulness; for this reason eye-drill for five minutes preceding a les-son in reading is advisable.

The child repeats the question asked: that is an act of imitation through the ear; try if he has good faculty in imitation of your movements through his eyes, which may afford a useful mode of training.

Translation of mental states from teacher to pupil, is largely effected by imitation of the visible expression seen in the teacher by the pupil. The appearance of strength, fatigue, or quiet mental attention in the teacher is imitated by the children, thus placing their brains in a similar attitude. Truly, the study of physiology does not lessen our moral responsibilities.

There is one item in imitation I wish to draw attention to. After telling the child to do as you do, raise your right hand: probably the child will raise his left, which is opposite to your right, in place of doing as you do; I believe such mode of copying should be checked in older children as being inaccurate. The principle of imitation extends to the smallest details; in teaching speech the pupil should look fixedly at the movements of the teacher's mouth, and imitate them as well as the sounds produced. To bring about such accurate imitation it is necessary to cultivate in the child the habit of fixing the eyes on the object he is told to look at.

Defect of memory in common matters, such as where to find books and things, very commonly depends not upon a brain-fault or defect so much, as not turning the eyes to look at the object, when putting it away. Losing things, especially dropping them unconsciously, is common in children with much spontaneous finger-movement; if the fingers open, the object falls; it is not seen and is forgotten.

Memory, whether as to where an object was last placed or as to past events, or memory of a lesson

learnt, depends upon two conditions in the brain : (1) a
sufficiently deep impression at the time the object or
the lesson page were seen, and (2) the re-activity of the
brain-centres. Defective action in the more purely
mental processes may depend upon not looking well
at the lesson to be learnt; trying to repeat it after
once reading, instead of reading it two or three times :
it is well to tell each child, how many times to
read the passage rather than simply to tell him to
learn it.

It will be interesting to trace the physiological principles involved in some of the tests of mental ability,
that have already been suggested and illustrated.

Among other principles involved are : —

Spontaneity of action.

Control of action through eye.

Control of action through ear.

Action coördinated by present impressions.

Action coördinated by past impressions in past —
results of training.

Repetitive uniform action in movement, and in expression of thoughts.

A spreading area of action — more objects of thought
expressed.

Diminishing area of action — some objects of thought
dropping out of memory as the examination proceeds.

Loss of coördinated action — as your examination
proceeds — Fatigue.

Association of pre-arranged acts — in movement and games or combined in expressing thoughts — Thinking, Logic.

Good or indifferent mental action in such points may be found; and corresponding to each may be seen similar good or indifferent motor action, as explained in speaking of the nerve-signs of brain-action.

These points are briefly given as a means of possibly starting on a well-arranged plan of training the individual child. It will also be found that, if the kind of motor action seen in the child does correspond with what you find on mental examination, you are enabled to form a judgment much more rapidly; agreement of results of the two methods of examination forms a basis for a well-grounded opinion.

It may be convenient to tabulate methods of mental examination in school, indicating the principles involved.

The pupil reads aloud. He is impressed through his eyes and by the sound of his own voice. Testing his accuracy of sight impression; he may correct his mistakes as he hears his own words.

The pupil reads to himself quietly. He is impressed through his eyes only. Testing accuracy in movements of his eyes and impressions received by sight.

The teacher reads to the pupil. His impression is received by sound and by sight of expression in the teacher whom he tends subsequently to copy, as in lip reading. Testing imitative faculty of expression.

The pupil recites from memory. Retentiveness.
Testing memory following impressions through eyes
and ears, and the faculty of expression in good speech.
Recitation may be better if he has seen and heard
teacher reading.

The pupil talks of the passage read. Your leading
questions draw out the expression of the pupil's
thoughts. Testing the mental impression he received
through his senses, and his faculty in connecting
thoughts and expressing them in words and gesture.

Class recitation of the passage read. Produces on each
pupil a rapid impression of the environment. Testing
capability for class working without excitement and
mental confusion.

Repeated recitation of passage pupil knows best. If
improved at second trial, he shows power of adhesion
of ideas and memory.

Answers to general questions on the passage. Testing
trained habits in thinking and expression.

Your mental examination thus conducted will bring
under observation children in whom what you see and
hear corresponds with their mental status, and may
indicate what to do for them. Repeating the question
is pure imitation by sound: try and use this imitative
faculty. Mental confusion is often accompanied by
extra-movements and a spreading area in visible action:
try and produce well-regulated movements in physical
exercises. Forgetfulness and bad memory may result

from inaccurate seeing and hearing. Inaccuracy in dictation and in transcription may depend upon defective hearing and seeing respectively, or upon faulty eye-movements. Children are often called silly, who speak in disjointed sentences not adapted to the circumstances, especially if this is accompanied by extra and fidgety movements or giggling; while others show simple mental confusion, and when addressed in the afternoon, saying, "good morning" or "good evening," or even "good-bye." Other children get red in the face and turn away or look awkward or confused when spoken to; they should be taught some form of social salute on meeting a friend and even how to shake hands. A purely imitative child puts out his left hand to meet your right hand unless taught otherwise.

CHAPTER VIII

WE have considered how to observe and describe a child in his body and as to his brain-action; as well as the points to be noted, indicating a sub-normal condition. I shall now describe various conditions seen in children, some of which are signs of a healthy body and brain, while others must be looked upon as faults or conditions of disturbance, to be removed, if possible, by care and training. The presence of some fault in a child does not necessarily show him to be either a weak child, or wanting in mental power. Certain types of childhood will be described to help us in speaking of the training adapted to different classes of children.

The most interesting conditions of the child's brain are the faculties of mental consciousness, seeing, hearing, feeling, thinking, which make up the inner mind-life of the child. You will find that the movements, accompanying and expressing consciousness, are mainly such as are stimulated by circumstances acting on the brain (through the senses). If speaking to the child, or showing him objects, is followed by his handling them and speaking of them, he is said to be conscious; or, if he subsequently speaks of those things, he is said to have been conscious, when he saw them, because we see that his brain was impressed by the sight; again, if the child does anything you tell him to do (ear-mindedness), he is conscious. The only normal and healthy condition of absence of consciousness is in sleep.

Sleep is so important to healthy child life, that, though it may not be seen in the schoolroom, some of the facts concerning sleep are well worthy of your attention, and I would recommend you to look at and study children in sleep, when you have the opportunity. In sound, healthy sleep the child is unconscious; there is a general absence of movements, except those of breathing; if you speak in a low voice, no response follows, and on gently raising the eyelids you will see that the pupils are very small, unless you wake him, when they expand; but you have made no permanent impression on his sleeping brain, and next day he will know nothing about your observations. The absence of movement in sleep indicates brain-rest, nerve-currents are not being generated in the nerve-centres, at any rate not in great strength, passing to the muscles to produce movement. The blood is circulating in the brain and nourishing it throughout, its force being stored up for the activity of the next day. Tooth-grinding sometimes occurs during imperfect sleep and is an indication of brain-irritability.

Complete rest during an hour in the day is necessary for some children; the child may rest by lying down or reclining in an arm-chair with a story book; this is best effected after feeding, when the blood is rich in nutritive material for building up brain-tissue. Rest resembles sleep in the little expenditure of nerve-force, but differs from it in the retention of impressionability to the surroundings.

Strength and activity of brain-power are indicated by good balance of the body, a lively expression of the face, and good tone in its muscles and around the eyes, without over-action in the forehead, together with much spontaneous movement, chattering, and talkativeness. These signs indicate spontaneous healthy brain-action, ready to be brought under control, without being stopped, under your care, by impressions received through the senses and in imitation of your actions. Accompanying such indications of activity in movement, there are probably many spontaneous, disjointed acts of thinking; if you can guide these, you may effect good mental culture. You want to train spontaneous brain-action to mental work, and when beginning lessons, you naturally require the children to be quiet, that they may think and not to disturb the class.

You call the children to lessons, the class assembles, each child stands in his place; the body is upright, hands hanging by the sides, and all parts, including the eyes and fingers, are motionless. It is assumed that the children are healthy, showing signs of good nutrition, their faces having a lively appearance and changing expression; thus we know that the motionless state is due to your having stopped their movements, and not to exhaustion. There may be one boy who is not motionless; his hands and fingers move, the left hand goes into his pocket, his eyes move away from you, when you look at him, his head is not kept erect. Following the indications and signs seen in the boy, you empty his left pocket and confiscate the top and crackers, which prevented the signs of attentiveness.

Do not expect the motionless condition of the body to be quite complete, but observe what parts move. It is one thing to stop these movements, and another to hide them; and again, it is a different mode of management to give the hands something to do. I have seen a nervous man stand upon a stool in the middle of a large room and make a capital speech. As soon as he began to speak, he put his hands behind him, and they were no more seen by those in front. I walked behind the orator to see what his hands were doing; the fingers were working away at a great rate, as long as he continued to speak. In like manner, when looking at an attentive class in school, "full face," as they stand, with hands behind, apparently motionless, I have taken a "profile view," so as to see what the hands might be

doing. Do not say, then, that "fidgetiness causes inattention," but try and describe what you actually
see in the children; thus you may study the condition and its causes by the scientific method.

You see a fidgety child; observe the movements
which indicate the fidgetiness, note the parts moving,
limbs, hands, feet, either on one or on both sides;
look at the head, face, eyes, etc. Then, when thinking about the child, you recall other examples of excess of movement. The fidgetiness you observe is
a physical fact, a number of movements not controlled like those of other children; look to the antecedents, and notice under what circumstances the
movements are increased or diminished. The movements indicating fidgetiness may occur in healthy
children when exhausted, when long confined in close
rooms, or when wanting food.

Say, you are thinking about the methods to be
pursued with a boy who is often fidgety and pee-
vish. You observe the movements of the child which
indicate the fidgetiness, the parts that move, whether
hands, fingers, or feet, on one or both sides, looking
also at the head, eyes, face, etc. You may find him
apt to mutter and complain, silly and childish. Observe him carefully; all reflex actions are wrong.
Call him, and his head turns away; when you speak
to him, no reply comes; when you say nothing, out
come his complaints. His phrases are simple, dis-

connected, and like those used by a younger child. The boy is for the time reduced, or turned back, to the brain-condition of a baby. There are also some spontaneous movements, which are but little controlled by his surroundings. Look out for the signs of fatigue and exhaustion in such a child, noting whether exhaustion precedes or follows the condition described. Irritability of temper often results from previous exhaustion, and it produces exhaustion. This is an important point, to be decided in each case by direct observation; it will be obvious that your practice must be determined by observation as to which condition precedes.

As opposed to attention and a quiet condition of aptitude for mental work, we speak of inattention and fidgetiness. Some of the best-brained, quick children are almost always fidgety : though they work well, they have more spontaneous movement than others, almost up to the point of adolescence : such are specially seen among the quick children of the nervous type.

Inattention may be due to conditions in the brain itself or its blood-supply. Prolonged abstinence from food renders the blood poor; a heavy meal draws blood from the brain to the stomach ; a close atmosphere renders the blood impure. On the other hand, the brain may be fatigued from prolonged work : I suspect, however, that inattention is much more often due to other things impressing the child, not leaving his brain clear and apt for mental work.

Fatigue is indicated by the small amount of energy expended in movement, such action as occurs being more or less useless and performed only under a strong stimulus, while it may be accompanied by extra-movements, but useless acts. Thus the child lounges in an arm-chair and does not get up when told to, but fidgets and grumbles.

Among the signs which indicate fatigue, I may mention the slight amount of force expended in move-ment; there appears to be a lessened total of force passing from the nerve-system to the muscles. There is often asymmetry of posture and movements, seen in the balance of the head, the spine, and the hands. There may be accompanying irritability, much move-ment upon the slightest touch, or movements apparently spontaneous. As you look at the child, you see too little movement on the average, or occasional jerky movements not controlled by circumstances. The eyes may wander and not be distinctly fixed by the sight of objects around, the face is toneless, less lively-looking, less mobile; possibly there may be fulness under either eye. There is asymmetry of action; the fatigued nerve-centres being unequally exhausted. Spontaneous finger-twitches, like those of younger children, may be seen, and slight movements may be excited by noises. The head is often held on one side, the arms, when extended, are not held horizontal; usually the left is lower; the hand balances in the weak type of posture,

often again more markedly on the left side. The direct
effects of gravity determine the position of the body
to a greater extent than in the condition of strength;
hence, the spine is bent. If this condition tends to
pass on into sleep, the eyelids are closed.

Fatigue is not itself unhealthy; both adults and
school-children must learn to work, and fatigue naturally
follows; what is needed after healthy fatigue, is rest
and recreation, renewing the power of the brain. If, on
the other hand, fatigue lasts day after day, a more permanent condition of exhaustion of great importance may
supervene.

Case 20. A boy exhausted and very dull.

A boy, twelve years old, showed weak balance of the
hands, with lordosis; his face was wanting in brightness,
with fulness under the eyes, indicating exhaustion.
His speech was good, and he presented no defect in
head, palate, or body. The teacher called him an idiot,
who could learn nothing. I saw no signs of organic
brain-defect, but marked indications of exhaustion. On
inquiring it appeared that the boy was kept at work
at home after school till midnight.

Exhaustion is an extreme condition of fatigue, in
which movement is lessened. The face becomes toneless and devoid of fine mobile expression, the circular
muscle of the eye is relaxed, the face may be lengthened
from relaxation of its muscles and slight falling of the
jaw; the ordinary movements of expression are not ex-

cited by the ordinary stimuli, and such movements as do occur are slow and laboured. A strong stimulus is required to induce the child to hold out his hands, and then the posture is the feeble hand. Sighing and yawning are common. Speech is slow, and the tone of the voice is altered. In some cases, finger-twitching, especially of separate fingers, indicates extreme exhaustion and irritability.

Irritability is expressed in a child, when a slight noise makes him start; this is a reflex movement in excess, a reflex action, that does not occur in perfect health on so slight a stimulus. In irritability other stimuli, besides sound, may produce excessive reflex action; a touch upon the shoulder causes a sudden movement. Not only is the amount of reflex movement excessive and out of proportion to the stimulus, but the kind of movement may differ from that usually following such a stimulus in health. A child three years of age, when irritable, may turn away his head from a familiar object, or from the sight of his food, and say " No, no here the sight of the object, instead of causing a reflex movement of the head, eyes, and hands towards the object, moves all from it. The irritability of the nervous centres is indicated by movements in the opposite direction from that which the same stimulus would give in health. Besides these reflex signs, we find the voice altered; when spoken to, he may answer sharply; the motor force, generally, is lessened and irregular; the kind, twitching irregular movements are not uncommon. Nervous children often show marked signs of irritability; the spontaneous postures assumed are those of fatigue, with the addition of slight irregular twitching movements. If this condition lasts long, nutrition is lowered and wasting occurs. Abnormal conditions in the body, particularly in the stomach, may render the child irritable.

Teachers have said that exhaustion in children is often due more to mismanagement at home, rather than to work in school. That may be so in some instances. Let me sketch a case for you.

Case 21. Girl tired in home life.

A girl, twelve years old, comes to school in the morning with too little spontaneous movement; the head is not held erect; the face is pale; the muscles around the eyes are relaxed; the eyes are wandering and not fixed or controlled in their movements by sights and sounds; the free hand is in the feeble posture. The attention is not readily fixed; she is fidgety and restless; such signs indicate exhaustion and irritability. We assume that the school is well arranged, and the work suitable. Later in the morning the child brightens up and works better, so that, at the close of morning lessons, she appears in better condition than when she came under school influences. Now, if the teacher knows, from questions put, or other sources of information, that it is not the school work, that produces exhaustion and depression, should the matter end there? If the teacher's opinion is founded on facts observed, would not any reasonable loving parent allow a friendly remonstrance or suggestion? If such conditions continue in the child, may she not exert a harmful moral influence in the school, such as may justify a stronger remark on the part of the school manager? Still, it cannot be expected that parents will readily listen to vague reports of their children, or to such as are not founded on precise and definite grounds.

The scientific observation of children has other advantages than the development of methods of public education; from the careful study of recorded observations we may improve the basis for research in physiological psychology.

All outward expression of mental states and mental action is by visible movements and results of movement; it is possible then, by analysis of such modes of expression, to determine something of the modes of brain-action, corresponding to mental states.

In sleep, or a state of healthy unconsciousness, we see that no movement is occurring in the limbs; the pupils are small; the movements of breathing are quiet and uniform; low sounds do not produce action or any subsequent expression. After such full deep sleep we see many spontaneous movements. We conclude that sleep is a condition of healthy rest, in which the brain does not receive stimulation from the outside, that its tissue is simply living and growing in a healthy manner, and storing up healthy force, which we see displayed in spontaneous movements after sleep.

Contrast this brain-state with that seen in a storm of passion. Bain says:[1] "The physical manifestations of anger, over and above the embodiment of the antecedent pain, are (1) general excitement; (2) an outburst of activity; (3) deranged organic functions; (4) a characteristic expression and attitude of body; and (5), in the completed act of revenge, a burst of exultation." Sir Charles Bell[2] gives the following description : " In rage the features are unsteady. The eyeballs are seen largely; they roll and are inflamed. The front is alternately knit and raised in furrows by the motion of the eyebrows; the nostrils are inflated to the utmost; the lips are swelled, and, being drawn by the muscles, open the corners of the mouth. The whole visage is sometimes pale, sometimes turgid, dark, and almost livid; the words are delivered strongly through the fixed teeth; the hair is fixed on end like one distracted, and every joint should seem to curse and ban."

At the commencement of an attack of rage, there may be momentary paleness : this is the best time for a chance of quieting the child. Then the breathing is seen to be quickened and the face flushes; the breathing is embarrassed, and the veins in the forehead, face,

---

[1] " Mental and Moral Science," 1872, p. 261. By Alexander Bain. Published by Longmans, Green & Co., London; D. Appleton & Co., New York.
[2] *Op. Cit.,* p. 21.

and neck swell out in consequence, while the lips are swollen and prominent. The eyes may move much, not being under control; while the hands are opened and closed, and gesticulate, and the lips may be seen to twitch at the angles of the mouth. The storm of movement may spread to muscles moving the larger joints of the limbs, the elbows, shoulders, and knees, as seen in biting and stamping. The order of occurrence of the signs is, first pallor, then flushing, and the congestion of face from impeded breathing; this is the order of events most common in an epileptic fit. The movements are first in small parts, afterwards in larger parts of the body. All this indicates a spreading area of brain in strong action, sending out force to the muscles; such brain-action not being under any kind of control from without. The exhaustion that follows corresponds with the large area of brain, that has been discharging motor energy, and wasting it. Here, as in other cases, a brain, not well under control, wastes energy that good guidance might have saved; good training is an economy of force to all, and specially in the weak children.

What good, what advantage, is there in these special modes of describing what we see? Modes of description here used are such as allow of comparisons being made. We translate abstract qualities, such as "joy," into concrete terms, such as movements, or conditions of form or development. We translate the terms, used to describe the abstract property, into other terms.

expression of the abstract. The term "happiness" is intended to indicate a certain condition of feeling, which we all, more or less, understand. The thing happiness is an abstraction; but if we can define an expression of happiness in man, we can deal with the material expression of happiness, analyse, and study it.

Having these descriptions before us, we can make some comparisons or analogies. In laughter, which is an expression of joy, or happiness, the angles of the mouth are drawn upwards; this is the very opposite to the expression of physical suffering. By defining the expression of the abstract thing, "happiness," in terms of motor signs, we find problems to deal with, capable of physical investigation.

All expression of mind and mental states is by movements and results of movement. You speak of intelligence, happiness, joy; for the purposes of scientific study, I would rather that you described the series of movements, which indicate these conditions, observing their antecedents and effects. Speaking of abstract qualities of the mind, you use, for the sake of simplicity, terms which indicate the aggregate condition; try to describe the signs you see, and to describe them in terms indicating facts whose causes you may deal with. It may be said that "fidgetiness is caused by inattention, and leads to forgetfulness." Each of these conditions is complex, and may result from complex causes; it is necessary, in scientific procedure, to try and analyse each, and describe it in terms expressing physical signs. Sometimes children get into a state of great mental excitement without passion; I have seen this during a recitation in school and will describe a case.

Case 22. Boy showing mental excitement.

The boy's speech became rapid, almost incessant, without intervals, the words were sometimes repeated; there was much movement in his face, and the pupils were dilated. The right foot was planted forward, the right arm raised free from the body, and the fingers were much moved, while the left hand rested firmly on the table at his side; his eyes moved much, as he was speaking, and the eyebrows were knit together; the head was extended backward, so that his face was turned upwards, and his eyes were raised above those to whom he was speaking.

Headaches are of common occurrence in children of school age; they are more frequently met with in girls than boys, as shown in the following table of 58 cases in my practice at the East London Hospital for Children.

TABLE VI

DISTRIBUTION OF CASES OF HEADACHE ACCORDING TO AGE

AGES	3-4	4-5	5-6	6-7	7-8	8-9		10-11	11-12	12-13	13-14	
Boys,	25 . .	1	2	2	8	2	1	2	2	4	1	0
Girls,	33 . .	0	2	3	1	2	5	5	4	2	4	5
Total,	58 . .	1	4	5	9	4	6	7	6	6	5	5

As a group these children present the general characteristics, described as common among nervous children. See Chapter IX. In five of the cases referred to above, the child described "sparks, colours, or other perversion of sight" during the attacks of head pain; sometimes distinct objects are seen, such as heads of animals or men; at night he may see "a lot of people coming to kill him," a policeman, or other source of terror. There is often a history of inheritance of headaches; among the 58 cases above, the mother suffered similarly in 24, and the father in eight cases; when the father and mother have both suffered from sick headaches, there is great probability that their children will also, and they should be trained and helped to bear pain. Headaches are often followed by sickness; the avoidance of fatigue and exhaustion is the best means of prevention.

Children with flat eyes (hypermetropia) may suffer from headaches, in part due to straining their sight in reading, from want of proper glasses.

Headaches in children are very common; they are of much importance, when accompanying the physical signs of exhaustion. I do not often ask children, if they have headaches, and place but little value on descriptions of their own feelings; but I constantly look for the signs of fatigue or exhaustion. When the child appears well nourished and there is no fatigue, headaches are of less importance. When I see a child presenting the signs of exhaustion, a toneless face, wandering eyes, fulness under the eyes, many points of asymmetry of posture, finger-twitching, and ground teeth, I put down such a child as requiring special care and careful education. Judge of the children by what can be seen in them, not by their description of feelings.

Case 23.   Headaches in a nervous child.

A girl, thirteen years of age, suffered from frequent headaches, during which she saw coloured stars, which sometimes preceded the head pain. She was a well-made but nervous child; her hands, when held out, balanced in the "nervous posture," and the fingers twitched, there was fulness under the eyes from relaxation of the muscles surrounding them. Three years before, she was disabled for three months by chorea. It is probable that the recurrent headaches will continue for some years; she must learn to bear them. It is not to be expected, that she can attend to her work in school or home lessons, when attacks of headache are troubling her. If training can remove the nerve-signs described, the child will be the better.

CHAPTER IX

Types of Childhood; and Groups of Children
below the Normal

The descriptions of Groups of children here given, and the evidence on the Propositions concerning childhood in Chapter XIII., are based upon the experience gained from 100,000 children whom I examined individually in schools. The results of that inquiry are published in a report[1] which affords a large amount of information concerning conditions of children.

Groups of children are classified and described, so as to enable me to present, in due course, the important Class of "Children who appear to require special care and training," to whom I would direct particular attention. It has always been difficult to define such children by what we can see in them; but it now seems possible to give a sufficiently clear description of the Groups of children included in

[1] Report on the scientific study of the mental and physical conditions of childhood, with particular reference to children of defective constitution ; and with recommendations as to education and training. Based on the Examination of 100,000 children seen in and near London, 1888–94.

Published at Parke's Museum, Margaret Street, London, W. Office of the Childhood Society. The Macmillan Company, New York.

that class, and to show the means of describing an individual child, indicating the points in which he may need special training.

The groups, here arranged, are of course arbitrary; in studying such groups the care of the individual child should never be lost sight of. It must be remembered that a dull child at one time classed as "delicate with abnormal nerve-signs" may another year be classed as "dull without defects," if the care taken has been accompanied by successful results; then we may hope that further mental training may make him a bright child, or average in mental power. The plan of describing children on schedules, or their defects on the cards, will keep before you the individual and the points in his case, to which attention should be directed; while the successive sched ules of the same child taken at different dates will show the progress made.

Normal Children. — From the school point of view, children may be classed as normal, if not found to be dull and backward for their age in lessons and in mental ability; while to observation they present the signs of healthy development in body, in nerve-signs, and in nutrition. Of course such children differ in individual characteristics, and in some of the general conditions described in Chapter VIII Again, some are above the average in their type of perfection in development of physical and mental power. Thus "Normal children" includes, as a group, all children not presenting any visible defect in development, nutrition, or physical condition, with no abnormal nerve-signs, and not found by the teachers to be dull or backward mentally.

I suppose there is no such being as "a perfect child," but it may assist to form a useful mental ideal, if we realise the characteristics necessary to a perfect type of childhood. His body must be well proportioned, the head of good size and well shapen, with each feature well made; while the stature and nutrition of the body reach a normal standard. (See weight and height.) Sight and hearing should be perfect. The signs of brain-action must be good in the movements seen, with sufficient spontaneity of action according to age; expression lively, speech clear and distinct, while, on mental examination, he must show intelligent appreciation, judgment, and a proper use of words in language, expressing thought and the faculty of thinking and remembering. The physiologist will require to know more than this before classing him as of a perfect type, and will inquire as to his ancestry and inheritance through each parent, as to what stock he comes from and the life-history of his collateral relations, brothers, sisters, and cousins. Habits in social life, and the development of some taste and enjoyment of healthy pursuits add further indications of a probable success in life.

A NORMAL CHILD

SCHEDULE FOR REPORT ON A SCHOOL CHILD

Number 24. *Name.* John Smith.
Age last birthday. 9 years. *Place in School.* Standard V

A. **Body : Development, features, etc.**

Head. Circumference 21.5 inches; transverse 13 5, antero-posterior 13 inches. Well shapen. No ridges or bosses.

Face. Eye-openings wide ; mouth of good size, lips well cut.

Ears. Well shapen, complete in all parts; not outstanding.

Nose. Bony bridge of nose well developed.

Palate. Sufficiently broad ; well shaped. Teeth not crowded.

Growth. Good ; height 51 inches. Light hair, fair complexion.

B. **Nerve-signs : Postures, movements, action. Expression.**

General balance of body. Stands well, feet together, legs straight and knees not bent, body erect.

Expression. Bright and changeful. An intelligent looking face.

O. Oculi. Good tone about eyelids ; no bagginess of under-lids.

Eye-movements. Fixes eyes well ; they follow a moving object accurately.

Head-balance. Head held well up.

Hands. Balance straight on level with shoulders ; fingers steady.

Response active and accurate. Sight and hearing good.

C. **Physical Health and Nutrition.** Healthy and well nourished. Weight 60 lb. Good colour in face and lips.

> **School Report.** A good child : is bright and intelligent. Recites well, quick at arithmetic, is rather high in school for age. Attendance regular.

> **Report on Child.** A healthy, well-made boy : he seems well trained in action of body and in mental power. He is likely to profit by higher education when old enough.

Date.

There is a class of children, commonly met with in every school, termed " nervous children "; I mean such as are apt to complain of headaches, are difficult to get off to sleep, bad sleepers, talking at night and grinding their teeth, while in the morning they are tired and not ready for breakfast. They are often bright enough mentally and affectionate in disposition, but apt to be irritable and passionate and too emotional. There are children who are delicate without having any disease; who are never laid up with any definite illness, but they are not strong, cannot walk far without getting tired; some days they are too tired to do anything and must rest; capricious in appetite, yet sometimes ravenous, but losing weight. A typical nervous child is generally well made in body, with a good head and well-cut features, a fine skin and light complexion; she may be tall and rather thin, with subnormal body weight. In the nerve-signs we see indications of weakness and over spontaneity.

The general balance of the body, as the child stands, is usually asymmetrical, with the head slightly drooped and inclined to one side ; while the spine is perhaps bent a little to one side, with unequal shoulders, and the feet unequally planted. The eyes wander much, in place of being directed to objects and fully controlled through sight and a spoken word. In the face, expression may be somewhat diminished, with fulness under the eyes indicating fatigue. When the hands are held out in front, asymmetry in balance of the arms is frequent, the left hand usually being held lower, while the " nervous hand-posture " is marked more on the left than on the right (see Fig. 6). As the hands are held out, the shoulders and upper part of the spine move backwards with an increased curve of the forward bend in the loins (lordosis), as a compensation in balance owing to weakness of the back muscles.

The fingers probably show twitching movements, if they are held separate from one another, so as to be free to move.

These signs show weakness, with over-mobility, and, if the condition is accompanied by a body-weight falling month by month or week by week, the child may, if overworked or if placed under mental stress by circumstances, or if frightened, pass on to the state of chorea. In mental habit such children are usually quick in learning, talkative, playful, and often laughing; in social life, they are gregarious, seeking one another's company, and, as they are usually imitative, may prove a source of mental excitement to one another. On looking further at such a child, you will probably find that the face is the best nourished part of the body, the limbs being thin; the teeth are very likely flattened at their tips from the constant habit of tooth-grinding. Appetite is very variable; these nervous children are very difficult to feed; at times appetite fails much, and again at another time they are voracious though they may still lose in weight. The care of such children will be referred to in Chapter XII.

Card showing the defects observed in a nervous girl as described above, and given in Schedule 25.

A NERVOUS CHILD

Number 25.   *Name.* Sarah Jones.
   Age last birthday. 12 years. *Place in school.* Standard VII.

A. **Body : Development, features, etc.**

> *Head.* Circumference 21.5 inches; forehead wide and well shapen.
> *Face.* Eye-openings large ; features well proportioned.
> *Ears.* Normal.
> *Nose.* Normal ; lips usually closed.
> *Palate.* Normal.
> *Growth.* Rather tall for age ; rather slightly built. Height 57.5 inches.

B. **Nerve-signs : Postures, movements, action. Expression.**

> *General balance of body.* Attitude asymmetrical : left shoulder lower than right, feet not equally planted.
> *Expression.* A little dull, and wanting in changefulness.
> *O. Oculi.* Fulness under eyes ; this disappears momentarily in smiling.
> *Eye-movements.* Eyes wander, but fix on an object if she is told to.
> *Head-balance.* Slightly drooped and inclined to left.
> *Hands.* Left balances lower than right, each is in the "nervous posture," especially marked in left. Separate fingers twitch.
> When hands are held out, the shoulders fall backward and the spine is bent forward at the loins (lordosis).

C. **Physical Health and Nutrition.** Rather thin and pale. Weight 75 lb.

School Report. Quick at lessons ; recites well. Talkative in school, playful and often laughing. Is fond of the society of other children like herself.

Report on Child. This may be said to be a nervous child : well made in bodily development, but rather under weight for her height ; though quick and bright mentally, she shows so many abnormal nerve signs that, unless she is brought under better control, she is likely to become an hysterical girl after leaving school at fourteen years. She needs careful training in physical exercises to remove each fault in detail.

M

CARD: SHOWING THE DEFECTS OBSERVED IN A NERVOUS GIRL, AS
DESCRIBED IN SCHEDULE 25

School............... Card No...........

Sf¹........VII...... Reg. No. .. 25....   GIRLS.

Age ....12......   .... Spl. Rep¹............

A	DEVELOPMENT DEFECTS	47	~~O. oculi lax~~	
a 1	CRANIUM	48	~~Eye-movements~~	
2	Large	49	~~Head-balance~~	
3	Small	50	Hand weak	
4	Bossed	51	~~Hand nervous~~	
5	Forehead	52	~~Finger twitches~~	
6	Frontal ridge	53	~~Lordosis~~	
		h 54	OTHER NERVE-SIGNS	
b 11	EXTERNAL EAR			
c 12	EPICANTHUS	**C**	~~NUTRITION~~	
d 13	PALATE	**D**	DULL	
14	Narrow	**E**	EYE-CASES	
15	V-shaped	64	Squint	
16	Arched	65	Glasses plus	
17	Cleft	66	Glasses minus	
18	Other types	67	Myopia, no glasses	
e 19	NASAL BONES	68	Cornea disease	
f 20	GROWTH SMALL	69	Eye, lost accident	
g 21	OTHER DEVELMT. DFTS.	70	Eye, lost disease	
B	~~NERVE-SIGNS~~	**F**	RICKETS	
43	~~General balance~~	**G**	EXCEPTIONAL CHILDREN	
44	~~Expression~~	*i* 82	CRIPPLES	
45	Frontals overact			
46	Corrugation		A ~~B~~ ~~C~~ D E F G	

Dull and Backward Children. — In the Report on School Children [1] all pupils were included in this group whom the teachers reported as dull or below the average in ability for school work ; by far the largest number of them were first noted on account of points observed below the normal in development, nutrition, or in nerve-signs ; a much smaller number were presented by the teachers as dull who, to my observation, did not present any outward signs of defect.

Dull and backward pupils are to be found in every school or collection of children. A child slow or backward for his age in knowledge and in trained mental ability is not necessarily wanting in brain-power or a defective child.

A boy may present a good type in each class of points observed, except his mental ability : while he can read and write fairly well and do simple sums, he may be unable to make any calculation in his head or to answer any questions, requiring memory and connected thought. Still he may be strong, healthy, quick to see and act and know what to do at the right time, and display good traits of character.

It may prove interesting to the reader and valuable for statistical purposes to quote the percentage of the boys and girls amongst 100 children, according to the average obtained. [2]

Taking 100 dull boys and 100 dull girls, we find

[1] *Op. cit.*, p. 154. [2] See p. xiii.

Among children seven years and under : 45 boys, 55 girls have developmental defects ; 49 boys, 44 girls have nerve-signs ; 23 boys and 30 girls are delicate. Note the large proportion of young dull girls that are also delicate.

Among children eight or ten years old : 43 boys, 42 girls have developmental defects ; 63 boys, 56 girls show nerve-signs ; 14 boys and 16 girls are delicate.

Among children eleven years and over : 38 boys, 35 girls have developmental defects ; 59 boys, 56 girls present nerve-signs ; and 7 boys and 10 girls are delicate.

These facts concerning the common association of defects afford explanation why children are seen so differently from different points of view, by the earnest teacher and the equally well-meaning parent. The teacher finds the child dull and backward; the mother sees the nerve-signs and indications of delicacy. A scientific description of the facts seen indicates both points of view.

A DULL AND BACKWARD BOY

Number 26.   *Name.* Edward Baker.
  Age last birthday. 11 years.   *Place in school.* Standard II.

A. **Body : Development, features, etc.**

> *Head.* Large, circumference 22.0 inches, frontal bosses.
> *Face.* Features coarse, none deformed.

Ears. Both outstanding ; large, no pleat to ear. They are red.

Nose.

Palate. Narrow, the upper lines of teeth meet at a straight angle in front.

Growth. Well grown. Height 54 inches.

B. Nerve-signs : Postures, movements, action. Expression.

General balance of body. Slouches, no exact symmetry of balance.

Expression. Bright, not very intelligent looking.

O. Oculi. Good tone.

Eye-movements. Can fix eyes well ; looks about by moving head, not eyes.

Head-balance.

Hands. Left held lower than right ; balance in feeble posture. Response in action rather slow and uncertain.

C. Physical Health and Nutrition. Good colour in face and lips. Robust. A strong boy. Weight 76 lb.

School Report. Does work in school, but is slow and inaccurate, and could not pass examination. Dull, but not defective.

Report on Child. Appears capable of work. Needs drill to quicken him and improve gait. A few minutes employed daily in class-exercises in imitation of movements and eye-movements would improve his brain-power. Possibly would do better with boys more of his own age.

A NORMAL BOY, BUT DULL

Number 27. *Name.* Tom Brown.

Age last birthday. 12 years. *Place in school.* Standard IV.

A. **Body : Development, features, etc.**

Head. Well shapen, circumference 21.5 inches.

Face. Features good and well proportioned.

Ears. Normal.

Nose. Normal.

Palate. Normal.

Growth. Well grown, rather tall and well proportioned in limbs. Height 56 inches.

B. **Nerve-signs : Postures, movements, action. Expression.**

General balance of body. Stands erect ; moves well.

Expression. Bright looks, active and playful.

O. Oculi. Good tone in all muscles of face.

Eye-movements. Looks steadily ; eyes follow a moving object well.

Head-balance. Erect.

Hands. Balance straight without movement of back, when they are held out ; action prompt ; speaks well, with clear voice.

C. **Physical Health and Nutrition.** Good colour, strong and robust. Says he cannot see blackboard unless he is close to it. Weight, 84 lb.

School Report. A general favourite, social, a good cricketer, but backward in school for his age, slow at learning, and poor at mental arithmetic. Has a bad memory, and is wanting in attention and perseverance. Not a bad boy.

Report on Child. A strong, healthy, well-made boy. No signs of defect ; he probably could do better at lessons if he tried, but he seems more fond of play than work ; if urged, he might do more. If we trust what he says himself, he requires concave glasses (for myopia) ; he should be examined carefully as to sight

Case 28. A boy small in growth, good at games, dull in lessons.

A very short boy, age fifteen years. Weight 5 st. 13 lb. (83 lb.); fairly muscular. Educated at a large boarding school during the last year, where he is in the choir; he plays the violin and piano. He is liked by the masters and his school-fellows ; he plays better at foot-ball than at cricket, and likes the gymnasium. His character is good, with a kindly disposition, both at home and in school. In the schoolroom he is very backward and cannot rise above the lowest form, though his education has not been neglected. He stands well, moves his eyes well, his action and articulation in movements are very good. The facial expression is a little blank, the muscles in the forehead over-act, and he is rather full under the eyes. His writing was fair, but slow. He could not distin... sh weights accurately. Speech was monotonous an s replies to questions long in coming out.

He appeared to be gaining but little intellectual culture, though growing in character. It was in school that he should have more to ... I earlier, give up Latin, and take more time in the workshop.

He was a good lad, capable of an active life, but not fitted for intellectual pursuits.

Case 29. A boy overworked, not deficient.

Boy aged fifteen years. Home in a British colony. He was solitary in habits, not caring to join in games or inclined to vigorous exercises of any kind. He had been taught Latin, French, history, arithmetic up to proportion, and some algebra, but he could give no clear account of what he had done in any one subject. He knew colours and could calculate a simple money sum. He was rather heavy, flabby, slow and inert in all modes of response; slow in dressing and in everything he did.

His head and features were well made, and speech good but slow; he presented a good expression and facial action, his hands when held out balanced straight.

He suffered at times from headache.

In his school-life he travelled by train 20 miles a day; he disliked his school and was not happy there. Returning home in the evening, he had tea, then prepared lessons, often working till 11 P.M.

There appeared to be no real defect of brain in the boy, but he had been over-worked and mismanaged.

Under observation it appeared that five hours a day was as much work as he could do at lessons without signs of fatigue. He required lighter work, he was not fit for

more than five hours' work under careful guidance, and
needed encouragement to active exercise.

With such a boy of inert disposition, it is better to
look out for the signs of fatigue, and if they appear,
stop work or change it ; but not to ask him if he feels
tired or has headache.

Case 30. A small girl, exhausted and placed too high
in school.

Girl aged ten years, said by the teacher to be one
of the dull ones. She did not present any signs of
defect, but appeared exhausted and nervous. She had
entered among the infants, and been moved up through
successive classes without due consideration of what
was best for her development.

Case 31. A backward girl, head small, eye-movements
faulty.

A girl thirteen years old was said to be a bad speller,
inexact in transcription, not bad in arithmetic, and not
generally mentally dull. Her head was small, but not
ill shapen ; there was a slight defect of the retina of
the eyes ; she did not move her eyes in reading, but
moved her head towards the words. Daily exercise
in moving eyes accurately was followed by improved
accuracy and better spelling.

Case 32. A boy bright at arithmetic, dull at Euclid,
did not look at the blackboard.

The boy was said to be industrious and not dull at
arithmetic ; but he could not follow a demonstration

Euclid on the blackboard. Observing the boy, during the demonstration, I noticed his eyes were fixed on the teacher, in place of the figure drawn on the board; he was frowning hard (corrugation with frontals over-acting) and evidently trying to remember what was said, but his eyes did not follow the demonstration of lines and angles.

Children Mentally Exceptional. — These children, while not necessarily dull and without brain-power, appear deficient in certain mental characteristics and in moral sense, such as habitual liars, thieves, and incendiaries; others liable to attacks of total mental confusion, a period of mental inaptitude or violent passion. Such cases are often described as moral imbeciles.

Some of these children are the offspring of insane parents or criminals. It is quite possible that some of these children were really epileptic or subject to *petit mal* (a temporary loss or disturbance of consciousness).

There is a distinction to be drawn between children intellectually defective and those "mentally exceptional." There are children who from moral rather than intellectual defects are unfitted for general training. Children dull from organic conditions are often solitary and unsocial, with defective expression, and it may be some mal-development; they may have some power of application and apparent attention, but gain little in education and are apt to be left out of all friendship by the rest of the normal children.

The children "mentally exceptional" form more serious group unfitted for general education These children show a distinct want of moral power; they are not solitary and are often bright and restless I do not know of any special signs or expression by which one can detect these cases.

Moral imbeciles who still are clever not uncommonly appear in the police courts.

Case 33. A clever boy; a thief and an incendiary

A boy thirteen years of age, mother died leaving five children, the father was insane; a brother twelve years old had tried to set fire to the house. It was given in evidence at the police court that the boy would often stop out at night and had stolen watches, rings, and a brooch This sort of thing had been going on for the past six years; if taken to a friend's house, he would be sure to steal something. There was not a lock, door, box, or window, he could not open. He was taken to stay at a farmhouse; one day, when every one was out, he took in a lot of "ragamuffins" and had an illumination in an upstairs room, and part of the room, it was found, had actually been alight. Since his arrest he had made an attempt to set fire to his own bedroom. His school-mistress said he was a very intelligent boy and in the fifth star

Case 34. A clever girl, but character bad, a bad inheritance.

A girl of twelve years, in Standard VI well healthy, quick, active, and clever in school defect observed, but a bad expression. Her father killed her mother, who was a drunkard. She was reported as clever at work, but an habitual liar and thief who had tried to set fire to the house.

Case 35. A boy eight years of age, bright and intelligent in appearance, had lost both his parents (the mother died insane). He lived with his grandparents. He was liable to such strong and sudden outbursts of passion as to be uncontrollable both at home and in day-school, and at length was withdrawn from school as unmanageable. When removed to the country, his health improved, and he became good and quiet, but when brought back to London, his bursts of passion returned. He had occasionally suffered from slight epileptic fits, and his younger sister also ; that was, in all probability, the outcome of his inheritance. When last heard of, the boy was neither being educated nor under proper control, and although at present harmless, and capable of being taught self-restraint, he is likely on arriving at manhood to be a social failure, if not absolutely dangerous to society.

Children Feebly Gifted Mentally. — These children are distinctly deficient in mental power, but should not be certified as imbeciles or "mentally defective."

No child is included in this group, unless it is believed upon both evidence observed and the teacher's report to be incapable of school work in the ordinary classes. It is not possible to define with exactness what physical conditions seen, as apart from mental tests, indicate the child as unfitted in mental capacity for the usual methods of education. There appears, however, to be a large number of "children feebly gifted mentally" with defect of mental power short of imbecility, but still with some deficiency.

These children may be described and reported on as to :—

(1) Mental tests; ability to answer questions, to make simple calculations, to read : as to speech and extent of vocabulary, knowledge of colours, coins, etc

(2) Signs of brain-action : response in movement and in imitation, fixation of eyes, want of changeful expression, frowning, weakness, and asymmetry in balance and other abnormal nerve-signs.

(3) As to development of the head and body or any developmental defects.

(4) As to physical health and nutrition

Sight and hearing should be carefully tested

No sharp line of demarcation can be drawn be tween the children feebly gifted and imbeciles, on the one hand, and as differentiating them from children simply dull and backward, on the other hand For practical purposes I think there should be two reports on such a child : one as to mental status, char acter, and habits, prepared by a teacher, with sources from the parents; the other by an expert, giving a physical description of the child, as he sees him

A FEEBLY GIFTED CHILD

Number 36.   *Name.* Adelaide Bennett.
Age last birthday. 13 years.   *Place in school.* Class of
                                       special instruction.

A. Body : Development, features, etc.

> *Head.* Small, circumference 19 inches, transverse from
> ear to ear 11¾ inches, antero-posterior 12 inches.
> Good shape, no bosses or ridges.
> *Face.* Features, except nose, fairly made.
> *Ears.* Normal.
> *Nose.* Bridge of nose wide and rather flat, or spread
> out.
> *Palate.* Narrow.
> *Growth.* Fairly tall. Height 58.5 inches.

B. Nerve-signs : Postures, movements, action. Expression.

> *General balance of body.* Slouching. Movements slow ;
> she tends to retain any attitude assumed. Imitation
> of movements fairly accurate.
> *Expression.* Fairly intelligent.
> *O. Oculi.* Good tone under eyes and in face generally.
> *Eye-movements.* Follows well an object moved, and she
> fixes eyes on an object.
> *Head-balance.* Not quite erect.
> *Hands.* Balance in nervous posture.
> She squints. The mouth is always open. Speaks fairly
> well, but utterance is thick ; there appears to be
> obstruction in the nose.

C. **Physical Health and Nutrition.** A little pale, but not thin. Weight 90 lb. Tonsils are not large.

School Report. Attends regularly a class of special instruction for backward children. A good child, truthful, honest; will buy and get change correctly. Counts well, knows value of money, reads simple words. Can do needlework and domestic work if urged to.

Report on Child. Is small headed and feebly gifted mentally, but appears educable; she is not troublesome, but wanting in spontaneous self helpfulness and probably in self-protection. She has benefited, and will probably continue to benefit, by daily training; she will need some friendly supervision and industrial training after leaving school. Medical attendance as to the throat is necessary, she probably requires spectacles.

Case 37. A girl mentally feeble, without speech, but with some social and moral sense.

Girl aged seven years. Small in stature and thin; weight 30 pounds; head rather small, circumference 19 inches, transverse 12 inches, antero-posterior 12 inches, fair form. Features and palate well made.

She does not run alone, but walks with very little assistance. There is a slight squint. There is very little speech, the child turns towards a sound; it is uncertain how much she hears, but she fixes her eyes on the face of a speaker, as deaf children do. I learned that she was not without the faculties of "moral sense and social sense." One morning she had pushed over a table with a flower on it, apparently on purpose; in the afternoon, when I saw her, she came to me, and without words pointed to the table, as if to tell that she had done wrong. She liked to be clean and tidy, and would help a little in toilet, and was social and kind with other children, patronizing them. She played much with a toy rabbit, and having seen nurse show it to a cat, did the same thing herself two days later. When custard and rice pudding were within sight, she made choice of the custard and ate it.

Mistakes are sometimes made; and children are thought to be deficient in mental power, in whom mental dulness is due to defective sight and deafness.

Case 38. A boy deaf, without speech, but educable.

A boy, nearly seven years old, was said to be uneducable; he had but little speech, otherwise there were no abnormal nerve-signs; he did not respond to a verbal direction, but was evidently deaf to a high degree. His imitation of movements by sight was good, and he made all his wants known; he fixed his eyes well in looking at any one or at an object, and when he handled objects, showed a varying expression at sight of them and made choice of what he liked best. The head and body were well made. His mouth was kept open; there was a large growth at the back of his throat, requiring surgical treatment;

this was attended to, and he improved much. The boy required to be taught to speak.

Case 39. A boy with increasing deafness, short sight and accompanying mental dulness.

A boy thirteen years of age, had been two years at a private school preparing for higher education. He had learnt some Latin and French, but was said to be so dull and backward that he had to leave the school. His action in movement was good: he could work out a money sum on paper, and the money values corresponding with coins; he wrote a good letter and expressed himself well in words. His body and head were well developed, as also his features He was very deaf and could only hear my watch at six inches; there was obstruction in the throat which had been neglected, and his deafness had increased in consequence. He was also short-sighted The boy did not appear deficient in mental power, but required surgical treatment and a pair of spectacles.

Children presenting Defects in Development. This group includes all children with one or more of the defects in development of the body that have been described.

Such cases are more frequent among boys than girls; the conditions of body observed may have no further significance; but, in many cases, other defective conditions are associated. Taking 100 boys and

100 girls with such defects as are described, we find according to the average obtained : —

Among children seven years and under : 23 boys, 35 girls also pale, thin, delicate; 36 boys and 40 girls being dull pupils.

Among children eight to ten years old : 16 boys, 22 girls are delicate; while 41 boys and 46 girls were reported as dull in school.

Among children eleven years old and over : 7 boys and 15 girls were delicate, whilst 37 boys and 51 girls were reported as dull.

Conditions of health may improve, as these children grow older; but an increasing proportion of them are found by the teacher to be dull pupils. To prevent such mental dulness occurring, these children should be recognised early in life, that they may be trained appropriately from the first.

Children presenting Abnormal Nerve-signs. — This group includes all children with one or more of the abnormal nerve-signs described.

Taking 100 boys and 100 girls with such signs as described, we find : —

Among children seven years and under : 19 boys, 27 girls also delicate; 43 boys, 47 girls being reported as dull.

In children eight to ten years old : 11 boys, 15 girls also delicate; 42 boys, 41 girls being dull pupils.

In children eleven years and over: 3 boys, 5 girls also delicate; 25 boys, 26 girls being dull pupils.

If, in methods of training children, more care were taken to prevent and remove "abnormal nerve-signs," the brain-condition of the children would probably be more receptive to mental training. The attention of school-teachers and educationalists might be directed to this object with advantage.

Delicate Children with Low Nutrition; Pale or Thin.
Such cases are more frequent among girls than boys, when we take the whole number of children in a school; when, however, we take only well-made boys and girls, excluding those with developmental defects, the proportion of delicate boys and girls is about equal. This fact may be important in considering questions of school method and arrangements.

Taking 100 boys and 100 girls, all delicate children, in school, we find : —

Among children seven years and under: 52 boys, 66 girls also presented some signs of defect in development of the body; 41 boys, 36 girls showed "nerve signs," whilst 43 boys and 43 girls were dull.

In children eight to ten years old: 51 boys and 50 girls presented defects of development; 51 boys and 51 girls showed nerve-signs; 40 boys and 40 girls were dull.

In children eleven years and over: 30 boys and 35 girls had development defects; 56 boys and 50 girls showed "nerve-signs"; while 37 of the boys and 35 girls were dull.

Delicate children are often dull and need training and teaching, as well as physical care in other directions.

No inquiries were made as to the feeding of the children, but probably those in resident schools, and the 10,000 in upper class schools, were provided with sufficient food. In all groups of schools it appears to be the "development cases" that suffer the most from low nutrition. Could we remove the frequency of these defects, we should probably have a smaller proportion of weak, thin, and delicate children.

The fact that delicacy and low nutrition are much associated with, and apparently caused by, mal-development, seems to indicate a constitutional or congenital flaw in the individual, often also associated with a tendency to brain-disorderliness and inertness. Such cases of low nutrition should not be neglected either in physical health or in education; we may wait too long for the child to grow strong; it is otherwise with conditions of ill-health due to temporary conditions or to disease.

It has been said that girls are more delicate than boys; inquiry and accurate description show that probably there is not more delicacy among perfectly well made girls than boys; when, however, girls are constitutionally weak, they tend more to further conditions of disturbance and disorder in greater proportion than the boys.

A DELICATE GIRL, HEAD SMALL, FIDGETY MENTALLY BRIGHT, BUT SUFFERS FROM HEADACHES; SHE NEEDS SPECTACLES

Number 40.   *Name.* Lucy Jankinson.

Age last birthday. 12 years.   *Place in school.* Standard VI

A. **Body : Development, features, etc.**

> *Head.* Small, but well shapen, without ridges or bosses. Circumference 19.5 inches.
>
> *Face.* Features well formed and in proportion to the head, which is small.
>
> *Ears.* Good.
>
> *Nose.* Good.
>
> *Palate.* Well shapen.
>
> *Growth.* Looks slight in build, but tall for her make. Height 57 inches.

B. **Nerve-signs : Postures, movements, action. Expression.**

> *General balance of body.* Rather over-mobile, a little fidgety.
>
> *Expression.* Bright, looks intelligent.
>
> *O. Oculi.* Rather wanting in good tone, but n t exact s full under eyes.
>
> *Eye-movements.* Fixation good, moves eyes well in looking.
>
> *Head-balance.*
>
> *Hands.* Held out well and promptly, right str g t left with three fingers bent back at kne s, s n "nervous posture." On holding out hands r t i s or throwing back the shoulders.
>
> When looking at a com, held 18 inches from face, ey s slightly converge.

C. **Physical Health and Nutrition.**   Pale and rather thin. Weight 70 lb.

Looks a healthy child, though rather thin and delicate.

School Report.   A bright child, works well in school; attendance regular, except when sick headaches prevent.   Complains that her eyes ache when sewing, but can see blackboard and reads test-type.   Is very fond of reading.

Report on Child.   A small-headed girl, bright mentally, but delicate, and is likely to remain so.   Eyes should be examined carefully; she probably needs convex glasses (for Hypermetropia), the use of which may help to keep off headaches.   Requires long hours of rest at night.

Dull and Delicate Children with Some Defect in Development and Abnormal Nerve-signs. — There is a group of *dull and delicate children* with abnormal nerve-signs, whose condition appears to demand that they should receive special attention; the physical report and indications of mental dulness agree in indicating them as unable to profit by the ordinary modes of training suited to the average and stronger children; they at the same time require more than ordinary care to prevent their failure in adult life.

A DELICATE BOY, DULL AT WORK, WITH SOME DEFECT IN DEVELOPMENT AND NERVE-SIGNS. NEEDS SPECIAL CARE AND TRAINING.

Number 41.   *Name.* Henry Harris.
Age last birthday. 9 years.   *Place in school.* Standard I.

A. Body : Development, features, etc.

Head. Circumference 21 inches. Forehead narrow and shallow.
Face. Features of face fairly proportioned.
Ears. Normal.
Nose. Normal.
Palate. Rather narrow.
Growth. Sufficient for age. Height 50 inches.

B. Nerve-signs : Postures, movements, action. Expression.

General balance of body. Rather listless, and asymmetrical in balance.
Expression. Fair.
O. Oculi. Good tone under eyes.
Eye-movements. Wander much, but can fix. Looks at words by moving head.
Head-balance. Straight.
Hands. Balance in "nervous posture," fingers twitch. When hands are held out, shoulders are thrown back and spine arched (lordosis). Slow and inexact in imitating movements.

C. **Physical Health and Nutrition.** Pale in face and lips ; limbs thin. Does not look unhealthy. Weight 50 lb.

School Report. Has been two years in Standard I., reads as a child of seven years. Does addition sums; cannot learn multiplication. Transcription fairly written, but inaccurate. Can learn poetry. Very dull, cannot get on.

Report on Child. Dull mentally, poorly developed in body, and delicate with listless irregular brain-action in movement. Would do much better in small class of special instruction, and needs careful physical training with some individual instruction. It seems likely that he will improve.

Epileptics, and Children with History of Fits during School-life. — In my inquiry these cases were asked for in every school. Any case with a history or indications of fits during school-life was entered in this group for what it may be worth. Epileptic children are not necessarily dull pupils, and the fits may be very transient, amounting only to a temporary loss or disturbance of consciousness (*petit mal*).

Many of these children are capable of school training and need occupation.

Epileptic children who retain intelligence are frequently left untaught, though their culture is of more than ordinary importance to prevent mental and moral degradation.

Case 42. Girl, age 13, Standard VII. Head and features normal, expression wanting; eyes wander and do not fix well; hand-balance feeble. Movements uncertain; she looks at others, before moving as told. Nerve-system is probably not sound; very dull in school, but improving. Has fits at home, none in school.

Case 43. Boy, age 11, Standard IV. General appearance is healthy. Epicanthis present. Expression wanting, smiles much, looks deficient in intellect. Speech indistinct and defective; did not talk till five years of age. Reported by his teacher as "very good and well conducted; very nervous; ability average in all subjects except reading, which is owing to defect in speech. Has fits in school."

Case 44. Boy, age 13, Standard VI. Head and features normal. Expression good; hand-balance weak, lordosis. A clever boy, conduct very good. Has epileptic fits both at home and in school.

Case 45. Boy, age 10, Standard IV. No faulty points observed in looking at the boy. He is intelligent, but has fits at home and in school, lasting some seconds, in which he falls down and kicks, has had as many as 160 fits in a day.

Case 46. Girl, age 8, Infant School. Head very small, 18.5 inches circumference, not badly shapen. Ears badly made in rim. Expression wanting, no response in action, will not speak. Thin and delicate "Does not speak, cannot read or write, but appears to understand some things said." Is mentally defective and epileptic.

Children Crippled, Maimed, Paralysed, or Deformed. — Those children vary greatly in brain-power, some are mentally bright, others dull. The conditions causing crippling are numerous; some are from disease of bones, others from paralysis. Each case needs to be considered individually in the school.

Children who appear to require Special Care and Training. — There is a small percentage of children, who in the aggregate form a considerable number unfitted, on physical or mental grounds, for the general education given in public schools.

A teacher of some years' experience may readily detect such children, but hitherto no fixed points (stigmata) have been recognised, by which it may at once be decided that such and such a child is unfit for general education.

Some difficulty has been found in forming any definition of this class of children. As arranged, it includes : —

"Children feebly gifted mentally."

"Children mentally exceptional."

"Epileptics."

"Children crippled, paralysed, maimed, or deformed, and the group of dull and delicate children who also present defect in development with abnormal nerve-signs."

I think that each of these children should be known to the managers, and that each case should be considered separately. It is not intended to imply that these children cannot be provided for in day schools, but they need to be provided for.

CHAPTER X

WE speak of children growing up and as passing on to adolescence, the period between childhood and manhood or womanhood. I shall here refer to some of the points you may observe in the older children, comparing their physical and mental characteristics with those of earlier childhood.

Spontaneous movement has been described as the great characteristic of infancy and early childhood; this markedly diminishes as years advance and is replaced by movements adapted both in speech and action by circumstances, expressing intellectuality and reasoning ; the child becomes less childish ; action should now be more fully under control of the senses, and of the impressions received, and should show the results of previous training. The nerve-system is so far built up (coördinated) by training and social experience that we expect lines of action and methods of thought and of speech, under given circumstances, to be much like that in other children of the same age and social position.

Social sense should now develop more strongly, showing character, avoidance of childish faults, more truth and accuracy in conduct and in word, with some thoughtfulness for others and appreciation of what has been done for the child in the past years and an awakening sense of responsibilities. At this age boys and girls differ more in some respects than in early years; they tend less to play together and begin to approach one another in social meeting differently, so that to allow sufficient freedom they separate more, which is not undesirable, if accompanied by mutual respect.

In boys and girls at this age the brain and nerve-system come more under the control of the feelings consequently wise control and guidance are wanted, while wider aspects of life and social habits may be appreciated which could not be understood earlier without experience. The children are now less childish and begin to demand respect as well as affection; at the same time they should learn to show respect and esteem for others. For some of the older children questions must arise as to their fitness and preparation for higher education after school, or for a business or profession and the duties of the coming years of social life.

Professor Key made observation upon 15,000 boys and 3000 girls at schools in Sweden, and found among the boys that there was a rapid increase in height and weight from the fourteenth to the sixteenth years among the girls the period of rapid growth or body appeared somewhat earlier. Dr. Bowditch's observations on children of American parentage, seen in Boston, show similar conditions of growth.   See Table III.

There is some difference of opinion as to the outcome of this growth period on general strength and form.   Professor Key has shown that, contrary to the opinion of many, it is a period of increased power to resist disease.

I think it will be found that the effects of such rapid growth in children differ for boys and girls, and vary with the different types of childhood as described (see Chapter IX.), and that among children with developmental defects or abnormal nerve-signs of the more enduring type delicacy and nerve-disturbance are apt to occur without due care to avoid them.   In this direction the avoidance of exhaustion and anæmia are most important ; practical wisdom consists in observing the individual child and being guided thereby in management.

I do not think that the boy or girl at the older ages of school-life, who is free from developmental defects of any kind and shows no abnormal nerve-signs or indications of delicacy, i.e. the normal child, is very likely to fall into ill-health or a nervous condition, if a wisely conducted training at school is continued.

Of the 100,000 children I have examined in school, 80 per cent of the boys and 84.1 per cent of the girls were normal and not reported as dull mentally.

It is, however, far otherwise with the children

who have some defect: anæmia, nervous disturbance, and hysteria may become manifest as adolescence approaches, especially in girls; when such become established, particularly if anæmia and nerve-disturbance occur together, a long period of ill-health may result

When consulted about a child as to the advisability of continuing school-life, I look for a good development and growth with the signs of healthy brain action and absence of defects: if nothing amiss is seen, I should advise continuance of regular study. If a course of hard work or severe study is to be undertaken, it is well to review the child or young person periodically, to see that no signs of fatigue or ill-health are manifest.

The desideratum at adolescence is to preserve and further cultivate health of body and of brain without in any way neglecting healthy mental power, which should continue to increase long after the period of adolescence. As adolescence approaches, observe the weight more frequently: look for any signs of fatigue after work and before commencing the day's duties, but do not question the child as to health. Continue physical training and require greater accuracy in movements as well as in speech, than at earlier ages. If paleness or the signs of fatigue or listlessness are seen, the cause should be inquired into, especially as to regularity in hours of sleep and as to feeding.

To understand some of the changes occurring in school children towards the period of adolescence, we may take those subnormal in some particular, and contrast (1) the boys at eleven years and over, with the youngest group; (2) then, the girls similarly; and lastly, (3) we will compare the girls with the boys in their advance during school age. For the facts here stated I refer the reader to Table VIII.

Boys at eleven years and over in contrast with those seven years and younger, are arranged in classes as before referred to; we shall see something of their progress in life.

As to the older boys with some developmental defect in body, more have abnormal nerve-signs or are slow, inexact, or disorderly in movement than when young; about the same proportion remain mentally dull or backward, but far fewer are delicate. These boys with badly made heads, or defect in physiognomy or growth, become less delicate in health with the progress of school-life, but the proportion of those with disorderly brains and mental dulness increases. It is shown in Proposition VII. (p. 248) that training directed to improve brain-action in movement lessens mental dulness; it is therefore clear that more attention to this matter is needed.

Among the older boys with signs of "brain-disorder-liness," i.e. *abnormal nerve-signs*, we find a smaller proportion of dull pupils than in earlier years, school training seems to sharpen them up.

Among older boys who are pale, thin, or delicate the proportion of those who are dull diminishes with school work, but still includes 40 per cent, and at all ages a larger proportion of the delicate boys are found to be dull mentally than among the girls.

Of the *Dull boys* in the older group a much larger proportion present abnormal nerve-signs than among the young; this combined with the fact that such signs of brain-disorderliness are always the most frequent accompaniments of mental dulness, again indicates how many dull boys might probably be brightened by further attention to physical training

Now as to the girls at eleven years and over, in contrast with those seven years and younger Of those with some developmental defect of body the proportion with abnormal nerve-signs has risen greatly, though the proportion of those who are delicate has fallen, the number still remains large, twice as great a proportion as with the boys while the proportion of those who show mental dulness has risen 10 per cent. This class of girls needs much care towards and during the period of adolescence.

Among the older girls *L.* *nutrition* is associated with developmental defect in a much smaller proportion of cases, than in young girls; their debility is presumably more due to conditions of environment.

o

still more than a third of these delicate girls approaching adolescence have conditions of constitution tending to low health.

Among the older girls who are dull mentally a smaller proportion of cases is due to developmental defect, and a much smaller proportion to delicacy; while a larger proportion are associated with abnormal nerve-signs.

We have now to compare the girls with the boys in their advance during school age.

Among cases with a *defect in development* in girls of the older age, this condition is more associated with nerve-signs, delicacy, and dulness than in boys, and such associated tendency appears to have risen from the earlier period more with the girls. These appear to represent many of the girls who have grave health disturbance as adolescence approaches.

Among cases with *abnormal nerve-signs* in girls of the older group, this condition is accompanied in a smaller proportion by developmental defect than with boys; but the difference is much less marked as age progresses. The proportion for children with abnormal nerve-signs who are mentally dull, is about equal for boys and girls at all ages.

Among the *Delicate children* the association with developmental defect is lower in the older group; whereas in infancy this association is more marked with girls, in the older group it is more marked with the boys.

Both boys and girls with developmental defect bear the effects of their environment badly, but the power of resistance seems to improve with years, advancing more with girls than boys. The proportion of delicate boys and girls who are dull remains much the same at all ages, improving slightly under school training.

Among the *Dull children* the proportion with abnormal nerve-signs is higher at the older age both for boys and girls, while the proportion of those who are delicate declines.

Having spoken of anæmia and hysteria as conditions of ill-health, not unfrequently developing at the period of adolescence, a short description indicating the signs of their commencement must be given.

Anæmia is a defect in the blood, in which it loses its colouring-matter. The red part of the blood is very necessary to health; it carries oxygen from the lungs to the brain and to all parts of the body, where the blood circulates. A person who is anæmic loses colour; the face and lips become pale, the colour under the nails is lessened and changes less when the nail is pressed; the patient becomes breathless and pants in going upstairs. The brain is much affected by the want of good blood; there is headache, giddiness, and drowsiness, a listless manner and inability for much active work. Hot close rooms, want of light, and ill-ventilation of the bedroom, as well as tight dressing, are among the causes of anæmia.

Hysteria is often combined with anæmia. The following points may lead you to anticipate a tendency to this condition. It occurs mostly in girls who are over-mobile, fidgety with their fingers, often moving about restlessly with their dress; the eyes may be restless and not under command, with the other signs described as common in nervous children. See Chapter IX. The balance of the head, the spine, and hand are usually asymmetrical, and the head may at times be extended; there is laughing in undue degree, on inappropriate occasions, and other expressions of emotion, the tendency to which may spread in the school among such girls. Expression of feelings and personal admiration, both in words and gestures, may be too highly wrought, while too much attention is excited by their personal appearance and that of others; there is a want of control over words and actions, with too few indications of intellectual thought and interest.

The tendency to hysteria may be inherited; there is often a predisposition in weak and nervous girls which can only be met by continuous careful training through many years; and it should be remembered that these children are often imitative, readily catching habits from one another. The brain-condition corresponding to hysteria appears to consist, essentially, in too great a governance of the mental state by impressions of the body rather than by the many things seen and heard. The mental state is too subjective, and the child's thoughts are concentrated on herself. Early detection of this tendency is important, that you may check its growth : avoid exhaustion as from late hours ; physical exercise and early rising are to be recommended ; try and improve any irregularities in movements or faulty postures of the body. As children advance in years, more work must be done leading to a moderate sense of fatigue, but signs of fatigue in the morning mean something wrong. As the child is growing up, educational training should be continued and should include wider interests, teaching thoughtfulness for others and at the same time the principle of self-control and some obedience to the laws of health, which in part replace the arbitrary submission to control looked for in early childhood. If at adolescence there be any depression, lassitude, and weakness, this should not be met by the use of alcohol, tea, or other stimulants.

CHAPTER XI

The Care of Children and Their Training

All knowledge obtained as to the physical and mental life of children, and the constitution of the individual child, should have a useful influence on the care and training of childhood. Observation and thought will enable teachers to gain a wide experience, and arrange their method in education so as to be the best available for building up mental faculty and good habits, while imparting the instruction necessary for the pupils.

A good deal has already been said about types and groups of children, and conditions in the child as you see him; these considerations show that the classification and arrangement of children in the schoolroom is worthy of attention. The pupils should be seated conveniently for the teacher's observation in an appropriate light; you cannot properly see a child's face and expression if he stands with a window behind him, and he cannot properly see your facial expression and action in teaching articulation unless your face is well lighted for his view.

An age-basis of classification in the schoolroom has largely been used, but it is far from satisfactory, and should be modified by a reasonable consideration of the intelligence, attainments, physical development, and brain-power of the children; if rigidly adhered to, the age-basis of classification may lead to very unsuitable grouping.

Children exert much influence upon one another through imitation; usually good results therefrom, but it is not so always; the advantage of this interaction among the pupils is one reason why they should be encouraged to play in games, and seek each other's society out of school hours. This concerns classification in the schoolroom; examples may be given where such influence is not for good. Excitable children, and those described as of the nervous type, are gregarious, seeking one another's society, and they are mostly imitative, increasing one another's fidgetiness with a tendency to inattention and too much laughter, unless they are separated in their school places. Children of the same family often show similar tendency to the same modes of action and the same faults, owing to similar inheritance. Thus, for instance, a child of the nervous type, one who stammers, or is inclined to be hysterical, should not be in contact with his brothers and sisters only, or with others of similar constitution, but is benefited by mixing with other classes of children, who in turn may be quickened by his action. Do not, if possible, place imitative pupils together who are ill-mannered or profane; it may be by contact with others they will better manners and more useful words, displacing the bad words they hear elsewhere: these children may perhaps be better placed among children rather dull, but good and less imitative.

I believe that the physical and mental health of the brain is promoted in all children by training wisely conducted; this in earlier years should largely consist in training movements such as bring about the faculty of coördination; a brain whose faculty for coördinated movement is built up under the stimulus of a good environment, mental and physical, works better in after years under the stress produced by adverse conditions.

In recommending early training for children as a physical means of brain-culture, I would insist on the avoidance of fatigue. The face may begin to lose expression, the lips and face become a little pale; there may be some loss of tone or fulness under the eyes. The tired child does not balance the head erect or the hand straight, and irregular movements may be seen. Spontaneity of movement, especially of the fingers, eyes, and small parts, is the character of healthy brain-action up to, say, seven years of age, and often much longer.

Spontaneity of action among the brain-centres is the fundamental faculty upon which good action and good mental power are grafted; this principle should always be remembered in brain-culture.

When the child enters the Kindergarten, a primary object should be *not* to make him sit still, but to train eye-movements; get the child to look at an object and follow it by the movements of his eyes; never mind if he fidgets the while, as long as he looks at what you tell him to; get him to look before you try to make him think.

Training the power of attention and removing inattention and fidgetiness are fundamental to all educational training. When studying the dawn of mental faculty in the infant, it was shown that the first indications of what may be called signs of attention, are seen when a sight or sound momentarily stops his spontaneous movements; a further stage is observed when such momentary arrest of movement is followed by a new set of movements, and gestures are controlled and regulated through the senses (brain-coordination). When at the sight of a toy the infant's movements are momentarily stopped, and the head and eyes turn to the toy while his fingers grasp it and convey it to the other hand or to his mouth, we say the child's attention has been attracted; we look upon this as showing faculty for intelligence later on. Spontaneous movements are constant in infants and very young children, the movements becoming less spontaneous and more under control by sights and sounds as growth and development advance. Analogous spontaneous movements are seen in young animals and also in all parts of seedling plants; much movement in well-nourished young things is the common law of organic life. This spontaneous action is what we want to cultivate, and when it is abundant there is the material to train. You must have action as the outcome of nutrition, before you can train and educate. Training is the process of bringing under control, bringing the spontaneity of the young into harmony with their environment. Doubtless it is true that this spontaneous action must be checked when you need the child's attention — that is a reason why you should not require "the attention" for too long a period together. If you have produced a good result, and no fatigue, spontaneous action will quickly follow the cessation of lessons. In play-time encourage spontaneous movements and cultivate them in games.

In early training we want to make the child, in accordance with his age, impressionable to the control of his surroundings and to place him in harmony with them ; hence the usefulness of organised play and well-arranged physical training of the brain. We want to cultivate the spontaneity of the child's brain-action, to regulate but not to stop it. Before trying altogether, to stop the fidgetiness which you observe, note if mental action accompanies the movement and see if the child be exhausted. Some children are always fidgety and inattentive, others only at times ; this may be due to physical causes acting temporarily, such as want of food or fresh air. Commencing chorea may be mistaken for mere fidgetiness, but is usually seen on one side of the body more than the other. There may be an appearance of inattention without any real mental fault; as when short sight prevents a child from seeing the blackboard or diagram or when dull hearing gives him but a faint idea of the question he is asked.

We wish to exercise all the powers of all parts of the brain. This may in part be effected by cultivation of precision of movements to the word of command, especially precision in movement of small parts, such as eyes, fingers, etc. Cultivate the faculty of imitation in the pupil by making him do as you do, calling into action the same movements of parts as you do yourself. Drilling lessons have often been looked upon only as means of "getting up the muscles," and they have been used accordingly by the drill-sergeant with the result that, as in the case of athletics, the maximum of good has not always been attained, and harm has sometimes resulted. Children may imitate the sergeant not only as to his exercises, but also in manner and expression. A few words as to the physiology of physical training may help an understanding of the object. When a muscle, duly supplied with good blood, is stimulated to action, it grows. The nerve-centres of the brain which stimulate the muscle are affected at the same time, and tend to act on future occasions with more exactness and more quickly when stimulated by the same word of command. If the object of the physical exercise of the class be to drill the nerve-centres or separate portions of the brain, increasing thereby the quickness and precision of their action, then the brain should, as far as possible, be free to receive the word of command ; you must get the attention of the class and try to perfect the time of their movements rather than to cause strong muscular action. Leave the muscles free, have nothing in the hands when you wish mainly to deal with the brain-centres, use no clubs or weights, and let the hands be open. Arrange your exercises so as to produce movements in some definite order ; at the same time, let them effect but little mechanical work. Let the movements following your word of command be such as to exercise many groups of muscles. In the limbs, exercise movements of the large parts and small parts, and movements of the separate fingers in flexion and extension, as well as in the lateral direction.

Each group of movements is due to the energy of a brain-centre, and these may be controlled to harmonious order of action by your exercises. Some very beautiful exercises with balls have been used, which tend, not only to regulate and quicken the effect of sight upon movement, but also to exercise the power of accommodating vision as the eye follows the ball. I think that this subject of drilling the various parts of the brain is well worthy of more serious attention than it has received. Well-managed exercises are most useful for nervous and slow children, exhaustion always being avoided. The child's mental processes may be too slow and limited in number; then try not only to quicken them, but, also, to quicken the capacity of the brain, for producing all movements and the interaction of the ear, the eye, and the hand, as in games.

There are two kinds of results of good training, - absence of abnormal nerve-signs, and absence of mental dulness; both results depend, in part, upon the child-material collected in the school. The normally made children should not present abnormal nerve-signs, an l in those of defective development much may be done to remove them — this is the ideal perfection of training.

Exercises in physical training may be adapted to the peculiarities, or the faults, in the child, as shown in his movements. Exercises with the hands in imitation of your movements and balance may be used systematically on a fixed plan. I referred to this in speaking of the examination of imitative power in Chapter VII, and will now go into more detail as to method of procedure.

As before, let *A*, represent the thumb; *B*, the index finger; *C*, the middle finger; *D*, the ring finger; *E*, the little finger.

Exact uniform repetition may be performed slowly or quickly; better be slow and accurate than too quick. Thus : —

$$A — AB — AC. \quad \text{Repeated three times}$$

with one hand, then with the other, then with both. After the exercise — return to the straight balance for a moment, and then drop the hands to rest. As the object to be attained is imitation through the eye only, after explaining what you want of the pupils, be silent while performing the exercise; see that the pupils fix their eyes on your hands, and do not simply work from memory. Be careful that no extra-movements, but only those shown, occur; no wandering eyes, frowning, side-movements of the head, shifting feet; get the action called for, only. During such exercises I have found the signs of fatigue occur, that may depend upon the details in your procedure. If the class consists of children seven to eight years old, as you stand before them on the floor or on a platform, your arms held horizontal are as high or higher than the children's heads, and they, naturally, tend to slope their arms up above the horizontal; thus raising their hands too high, and spending more energy than you intend, while the shoulders are probably thrown back in this unnecessary effort, with bending of the lower part of the spine (lordosis). If you sit on a low chair, on a level with the children, all this may be prevented.

When you tell them to imitate you in holding out hands in front, and you do it slowly, do not allow a quicker movement than you make; some children will shoot out their hands with too much energy, and this is often done with closed fists, or anything but a straight balance of the hands. Such action is analogous to the habit of some children of shouting, when answering in class; both are bad manners, an! a waste of strength. It is the exact control by imitation that best trains the brain.

A gradually increasing series of movements will be more difficult for imitation. Thus:—

$$A - B - CD --- E - AB - AC - AD - AE.$$
$$ABC. \quad ABD. \quad ABE. \quad ABCD \quad ABCDE.$$

This may be performed first with the right hand, then with the left, finally with both together

Many other similar exercises might be arranged, the series of movements becoming more complex

Eye-movements need training in all children till they have acquired the faculty of accurately an I steadily looking at objects and their parts Exercises in eye-movements may be conducted in various ways: tell the children to look at a small object you hold in your hand, and to follow it with their eyes without moving the head; they may then look at a ball as it passes through the air Eyes are more readily fixed by a bright object, as a bright coin, than a dull one; gold has generally greater attraction than silver. It is useful in difficult cases to use a small lamp; or employ a small hand mirror and a well screened lamp, so as to reflect its light on the ceiling and wall, which young children like to follow Again, you may name known objects in the room, or pictures, telling the pupils to look at each, thus quickening their movements; this may be followed by counting the objects with their eyes.

Training should also be given in estimating the weight and size of objects after the methods explained in testing mental ability. See Chapter VII.

I have thus far been speaking of exercises planned to train exact movements of small parts : such exercises train the power of brain in its finer faculties of coördination through the eyes, fitting it for the purely mental functions of thinking. These exercises may be fatiguing, in the sense that though the children may not look fatigued as the face is seen, after a short time of practise the movements become less accurate, then stop the exercise : this is analogous to inaccuracy from mental fatigue. Exercises of fingers and eyes may be dropped and the lesson concluded by movements of larger parts, the shoulders, elbows, hand exercises with closed fists, or allowing the fingers to be free or to move spontaneously and uncontrolled in the arm exercises. I believe it will be found useful if the class teacher himself will devote five or ten minutes a day to physical training of the brain as described, as apart from the general calisthenic exercises that may be given in the school.

I do not say much about drill, marching, military exercises, and the use of the gymnasium; each mode of training is useful as well as some form of free exercises on the lines of the Swedish system; these have been described by those who practise and teach them. All such exercises improve the muscles and growth; they promote physical health, a good gait and carriage, and general activity.

It must be recognised that though spontaneous movements of the digits are seen at birth, the larger muscles are more easily brought under control than the small ones, at an early age. With children seven years old and under do not expect very exact imitation of finger movements, but rather equal planting of the feet, good time in marching; use exercises for the limbs with the hands open, allowing spontaneous movements of the fingers to occur while the larger muscles are controlled in action.

The purpose of your physical training is to regulate and control the brain of each child, and the class as a whole; such exercises improve action, response and balance of the body, head, and limbs. A further object is to remove any abnormal nerve-signs present, and render the nerve-system strongly knit together that it may bear strains well in the future.

Probably, by careful physical training and exercises in imitation, you will succeed in effecting a good carriage of the body, and balance and action in the limbs, but you will find more difficulty in implanting a good expression of face, in improving the tone of the muscles of expression and, in particular, that around the eyes (orbicularis oculi), as well as in relaxing overaction of the muscles.

P

crumpling of the forehead. This leads me to speak of
dealing with the following abnormal nerve-signs : Expression defective. Frontals overacting. Corrugation.
O. oculi lax ; these are nerve-faults, in fact bad habits,
if you will call them so, but it is generally useless to tell
the child to look happy and not to frown or knit his
brows.

These signs in the forehead are overaction in place
of quietness. It may seem to you curious that the same
sign, the same muscular action in the face, should under
different circumstances indicate almost opposite conditions. These signs may be due to (1) too little mental
action or stimulus; (2) they may indicate a rather excessive amount of mental action or its results.

Case 47. In some institutions for boys where they
lead a monotonous life, and in an asylum of imbeciles,
horizontal frowning is frequent. In a Kindergarten I
was looking at a small boy with a dull face and frontals
overacting : when I spoke to him and asked him what
he was going to do, he seemed interested, and his face
became quiet but more expressive ; so also when he
began work, making a mat of coloured papers, he looked
bright. Sometimes just quietly looking at the child as
he looks at you is sufficient stimulus, and frowning subsides. In these cases mental stimulus does good : on
the other hand, hard mental work may cause these signs,
or at least these signs may accompany mental effort.
When a class is working sums on paper, or answering

questions in mental arithmetic, in some boys the eye-brows are raised and knit together strongly, a useless set of extra-movements accompanying mental action.

Thus, in trying to remove these signs in a child, observe whether they occur mostly when he is occupied or unoccupied, what you see will guide your action: the abnormal signs should be got rid of if possible. Too strong a light may cause a child to screw up his eyes and frown : coarse repeated frowning may be seen in a child otherwise normal when he presents signs of fatigue after work.

If the child has a dull expression, try and make him laugh, and laugh with him, not at him ; make a joke or tell a short story and set all the class laughing for a moment, to see if he will join in. Exercises involving an increasing number of movements may cause interest, and a little excitement, if there be no fatigue. Fulness and want of tone under the eyes often accompany a want of expression and occur frequently with headaches. It is removed in laughter, and if due to a temporary cause, the fuller tone produced by laughing may remain ; note the time of day when it is seen, and if it correspond with general languid action.

In the classroom of the fifth standard boys in a school at afternoon lessons I found nearly half the number of pupils looking full under the eyes. The school was not working at high pressure, but the m

was overcrowded, hot, and close ; more air and ventilation were needed.

Not speaking the truth, and petty untruthfulness
of word and action, must of course be reproved and
checked in childhood: I do not wish to put down all
child faults as mere physical weaknesses, but it may be
useful to see how in some cases untruthfulness is associated with conditions that may be removed by training.

A boy slams the door and then says he didn't ; or
you see his foot kick his neighbour, and he denies it.
The door may have slammed because his fingers
twitched and let it go or pushed it, and his foot may
have struck his neighbour from uncontrollable movements.   Before you are quite sure the action was intentional, look and see that there are no great number
of spontaneous movements occurring.   I have known
children punished on account of the inconvenience
resulting from the irregular antics of commencing
chorea.   A boy says he has learnt his lesson, but cannot repeat a word of it, having learnt the wrong one,
but being afraid to say so — he may be a child with
untrained eye-movements, and did not look accurately
to see the number of the page he should have learnt.
Such faults may not be intentional lies on the child's
part.

Case 48. A child at school had a sick headache
while writing notes of the lessons to be prepared at
home.   Looking at the note-book next day, several

words were repeated, and others omitted, while the whole was most inaccurate, though usually carefully entered; the hand-writing was also altered, showing a brain disturbance as the cause of forgetfulness

Some nervous children are very timid and liable to mental confusion when suddenly addressed, turning pale or flushing, not ready with any appropriate reply, and full of extra-movements when excited. If their mental confusion is mistaken for deceitfulness or untruth, confidence may be lost between the teacher and pupil : such children are often keenly sensitive to an injustice, or what appears so to them.

Case 49. A boy living with his friends, away from his parents, attended a day-school and was generally docile and good. One day he said at school that he had been told to go back early; this proved to be totally untrue, and he was punished. On another occasion, he told the master at school that he had a little baby brother and had received a letter saying the baby was dead and he was to go and see him. I showed the letter, which said nothing of the kind. This without further inquiry was apparently a second untruth. That boy was the son of a mother not of very sound mind; he had had a few slight epileptic fits, and sometimes saw — apparently really that he saw and heard — persons who spoke to him

Illusions are not uncommon among children and adults who have no unsound mind. A child may over and over again see an ugly man, a dog, or a wolf; such illusions may cause secret fear or they may not annoy him. Get the child if you can to tell you of what he sees, explain to him that they are only dreams; do not speak often of them, but do not avoid them.

Fixed mental impressions are important elements in mental life; some you may wish to build up, others you may wish to remove; the first thing is to discern their existence. A fixed and oft-repeated facial expression of mental anxiety not produced by the circumstances may accompany illusions; blushing not due to any visible cause may result from· a fixed thought producing fear or emotion. Find out if you can the source of the fixed thought that produced it; it may be some object seen that caused fright; epilepsy may follow fright or the oft-repeated imagination or calling back to view that dreaded sight or the mental impression it produced.

You may sometimes see a child immovable, apparently unimpressed by all around him, the eyes fixed with a stare. You conclude he is not thinking, as you can get no expression of thoughts from him. Such habits ought to be checked.

As to the management and training of delicate children: I wish in the first place to insist on their need of training and education, suited to their condition and their capacity; it is a mistake, only too common, to leave weak children to do nothing all day, hoping that they will grow stronger

The care of such children concerns management both at home and in school.

A detailed study of nerve-signs in the child will give assistance of scientific and practical value to those in charge of delicate and nervous children A card indicating the abnormal nerve-signs in the case (see Card, Nervous Child, Chapter IX) will show the teacher some of the points to be aimed at in physical training; further, a knowledge of the brain-disorderliness indicated by the signs will give a hint as to the modes of mental disorderliness likely to be met with in the pupil. Wandering eye-movements lead to inaccuracy in transcription and sometimes in arithmetic; children with twitching finger movements not easily controlled often have spontaneous thoughts arising, which lead to mental confusion and inaccurate answers to questions also interfering with memory. The child slow in all movements and slouching is apt to be dull in mental action till his attitude and response are improved

The description of the child points out as signs of brain-disorderliness : " want of facial expression," " listening," " frowning," " knitting of the eyebrows," the " want of control of movements," " protrusion of the tongue when spoken to," " lordosis," and " rabular and hand-postures." It is the teacher's part to try and also to remove each such abnormal nerve-sign and the brain-disorderliness corresponding, by presenting a good copy for imitation in balance and in action. Observing the circumstances under which each of the given signs most frequently subsides will help you to carry on brain-training concurrently with purely mental training.

Untrained children often grow up to adult age without their eye-movements having been brought under control, leading to habits of inaccuracy in book work : such children make very bad observers.

The mental training of delicate children needs to be carefully regulated. It is a mistake to leave delicate children untrained and uneducated ; such neglect often leads to hysteria in adolescence, weakness, inability to bear headaches without nerve-prostration and other inconveniences, and disabilities in adult life. Further, good training improves brain-power, lessens brain-wear, and lessens the tendency to mental confusion and disorderliness.

Spontaneous action in the higher brain-centres, both for motor action and for mental action, is very commonly found in excess in nervous and delicate children ; it is then sometimes said that they are precocious and should not do lessons ; these young brains are often well made, and will work, and may lead the child if left at home with nothing to do to fall into the habit of an amount of lonesome thinking which produces bad sleep and exhaustion. Such children benefit by a quiet regular school-life and association with

other pupils, in whose work and games they must take
their part.

As to the schoolroom management of a nervous
child, it is necessary to observe whether he is more
easily and quietly controlled through his eye or ear;
speaking to him may be followed by some extra-movements and fidgeting, whereas signalling or indicating
by your gesture that he must go on with his work,
or not talk, may be followed by quiet obedience.

I wish to encourage among teachers the study of
Nature's works, conditions of life as seen in plants and
animals — the child is a part of Nature's work All
the properties of the brain which give it the faculty
of expressing the action of mind are seen, in some
degree, in lower living things. The study of natural
objects, and their processes of growth, may suggest
methods for use in mental training. Suppose an
object lesson on botany. You want to use some piece
of Nature's work placed before the class, or better
still, in the hands of each pupil, as a means of education in observing and thinking, as a means of teaching
processes of thought and extending the mental capacity of the pupils, together with the cultivation of
accuracy of method — this is the desire of every scientific teacher. Observing is not necessarily thinking,
observing is receiving new impressions, thinking is a
series of brain-acts that may follow such impressions
Observation may, or may not, lead to thinking of

depends much upon the teacher whether the object lesson shall teach thinking or only observing. Impressions produced by sight of the specimen may be followed, after it is removed, by thoughts; descriptions given by the pupil are expressions of thought, and help to enlarge his vocabulary. Suppose you take some simple leaves not notched upon the margin, and speak of them with regard to their shape. You may describe them as oval, elliptical, ovate, obovate, lanceolate, etc., using a new term for every shape, that is, using a number of terms, one for every shape or ratio in the length of the transverse and median axis; in place of this you may indicate the ratio; say, let us consider the form as determined by the ratios of the axes, and do without a long nomenclature.

(oval) median axis . . length 3 ⎫ the axes crossing at their
 "   transverse axis . . . 1 ⎭   centres at right angles.
(elliptical) median axis . . . 4 ⎫ the axes crossing at their
 "   transverse axis . . 1 ⎭   centres at right angles.
(ovate) median axis . . . . 3 ⎫ the axes crossing at right
 "   transverse axis . . . 1 ⎭ angles ⅓ from the base.
(obovate) median axis . . . 3 ⎫ the axes crossing at right
 "   transverse axis . . 1 ⎭ angles ⅔ from the base.

It is unnecessary to go further into details. As to these two modes of describing form of leaves, the second indicates what you observe on looking at the leaf. There is a great difference between teaching science and scientific teaching. Let me give another

illustration of description of growth,[1] which may stimu
late more thought than the simple one given above
Look at horse-chestnut buds in different stages of
growth. During the winter months the inner parts of
the bud are enclosed by scales, or modified leaves ; as
these scales grow, the cells on the outer surface in
crease more rapidly than those on the inner surface,
and, as a mechanical result, these scales become more
concave towards the centre of the bud and envelop
it, thus affording protection from the weather and
attacks by insects. The young imperfect leaves are
closely packed within, and these also grow quickly on
their outer side, causing them to press towards the
centre of the bud. When spring-time comes with
increased temperature and consequent increased nutri
tion, changes occur in the ratios of growth — the inner
surfaces of both bud-scales and young leaves grow at
a greater rate than the outer surfaces, and thus the
curvatures are altered, the inner surfaces become convex, and the bud opens. How much simpler it would
be to say — the bud opens to the spring.' But the
detailed description teaches us to think ; it shows that
we must consider the individual parts of any living
thing when we want to know how it acts ; the ratios of
action in each part must be observed. We see the fun

1 For further examples, see Author's work, " Neat ms : M   :
Treatise on the Action of Nerve-Centres and M es of Gr a'   1:
Macmillan Company, New York.

does not open itself, neither is it a mere machine,
as the phrase is commonly understood. Warmth is a
necessary antecedent to the processes described ; the
ratios of growth appear due to properties inherent in
the cells composing the parts.

Having referred to different modes of giving descriptions of facts in Nature, we may use the principles put
forward as a means of analysing literature.   Let me give
two examples from " Nathan the Wise " (Lessing).

NATHAN

"The searching eye will oft discover more
Than it desires. 'tis as he read my soul.
That, too, may chance to me. 'Tis not alone
Leonard's walk, stature, but his very voice.
Leonard so wore his head, was even wont
Just so to brush his eyebrows with his hand,
As if to mask the fire that fills his look."

Here is a description of what Nathan saw in Leonard ;
the terms used are his stature and the various movements seen — a purely physical description.

CONTI

"This head, this face, this forehead, these eyes, this nose, this
mouth, this chin, this throat, this bosom, this figure, this whole
form, are from this time forth my sole study of feminine beauty "
(" Emilia Galotti " — Lessing).

Here is an unspiritual and corporeal description,
without reference to any movement or sign of brain-
action.

We will now take for analysis the following description of the condition of Achilles :[1]

> "Achilles heard, with grief and rage oppress'd ;
> His heart swell'd high, and laboured in his breast.
> Distracting thoughts by turns his bosom rul'd,
> Now fir'd by wrath, and now by reason cool'd "

This description we should find hard to analyse and translate into terms denoting what can be actually observed ; this illustrates the convenience of non-physical terms.

I have touched briefly upon many points, speaking of things as I see them. The great labour, responsibility, and honour of educating children is yours. The words of the poet remind us that :

> "Knowledge comes, but wisdom lingers."

It is not enough to give children knowledge ; you should be wise for their sakes, and to become so may find it well to study Nature in her works and the child as a part of Nature.

---

[1] Pope's translation of the "Iliad," line 251.

CHAPTER XII

Hygiene and Health Management during School-Life

I shall speak of children now from the health point of view, and deal with methods of cultivating healthy conditions in the school and in individual pupils, as well as preventing illness and the spread of disease. I shall bear in mind that the main object of this work is to indicate points for your observation in the children, and subject for thoughtful consideration. Advice may sometimes be conveyed to parents through their children, so that while you give attention to general points of health in the school, you may help individuals and at the same time spread knowledge among the elder pupils on practical matters of health-culture, which no formal teaching would impart, and thus inspire them with the desire for a healthy body with a sound mind. I shall speak of general points in health-culture, and of methods for early detecting and the means of preventing the spread of illness and disease.

A point of first-rate importance to health is cleanliness in person, in dress, in the air breathed, and in food. The air of any living-room should be constantly changed : the emanations in the breath are poisonous, foul air causes headaches, drowsiness, mental dulness, and diseases. In the schoolroom the temperature in winter should not fall below 50' F., nor rise above 60° F.; it is desirable that there should be a short interval in the middle of the morning lessons, that the windows may be thrown open widely and the air thoroughly changed. In any living or sleeping room the windows should be opened a little at the top, while a small fire helps ventilation by causing a draft up the chimney.

As a matter of school hygiene teachers should take notice of the early indications of illness or disease. Perhaps the most practical means of looking to these points in the children day by day, is for the class teacher to receive the pupils as they arrive and cast a glance at each child for a moment. If any child is thought to be feverish, the temperature should be taken by the thermometer, and the appearance of any rash should be looked for in the face and on the skin of the chest. Among common chronic conditions, that may be seen, I may mention discharges from the eyes, nose, and ears, diseases of the skin and the scalp; the dangerous diseases you may occasionally see those of the infectious fevers and diphtheria, while or St. Vitus's dance may develop gradually during attendance, growing worse day by day. Seen when speaking to a girl of her home life and asking after the younger brothers and sisters, you may be able to give useful advice.

I shall speak now of food and the feeding of children, their clothing, and the care of those that are delicate. Some mistakes are made among the poorer classes, more through ignorance and want of helpful guidance than through poverty; cheap food is not always economical, and the use of suitable food and proper feeding does not always mean more expenditure.

Milk should be obtained as fresh as possible and not kept longer than necessary; it should be received in a freshly scalded jug and placed out of the way of dust, covered with muslin or a sheet of clean paper, to keep out the dust: dust makes milk go sour, and the germs of disease grow rapidly, increase, and multiply when they fall into milk. In hot weather the milk should be scalded, if it has to be kept through the night; neglect of this in the summer may cause much disturbance in children.

Water does no harm to children, but large quantities should not be drunk when the child is overheated; many children suffer much from not being able to drink when they want to. If there is doubt as to the purity of the water, it should be boiled and allowed to cool before drinking. All children are better without beer or any alcoholic drink.

Bread should not be used till the second day; new bread is both indigestible and wasteful: broken bread and bread crumbs may be used for bread and milk or in puddings.

Fat food is very desirable for children. With bread they should take butter or dripping or the fresh marrow of bones; bacon, eggs, as well as fresh meat with fat, form very nutritious food. Suet pudding, made with equal weights of suet, flour, and bread crumbs, well mixed and long boiled, is nutritious and digestible.

Green vegetables and fruit in season are useful; the latter should not be used when at all decayed, as it often causes illness. The value of potatoes as nourishing food is apt to be overestimated.

Fresh fish and meat are of course highly important, but I have no space to speak of these articles of diet.

The habit of taking meals regularly at fixed times, never being late or hurried at breakfast, is equally important to good living with the kind of food provided; the meals taken at home with due order will give a better digestion of the food and better nutrition of the body and brain, than snacks of bread and butter or odds and ends of food taken irregularly.

The teacher — thinking of the future pupil — may upon occasion have the opportunity of advising parents as to the feeding of an infant: this matter is too important to pass over even if the senior girls are not well instructed on such matters as points of physiology.

Many of the troubles of early childhood in a town population result from the development of rickets; this is a condition of bad growth with bent legs and other defects which is largely due to giving babies farinaceous or starchy food under seven months; on the other hand, rickets may often be prevented and the child's health much improved by strict attention to healthy surroundings and proper and regular feeding.   At six months old a hand-fed baby should take two pints of milk in the twenty-four hours diluted with one-third water or with a little lime-water or barley-water.   No artificial food, containing starchy matter, or biscuits or bread should be given, at any rate till after the first teeth are cut. Great care should be taken to keep the feeding-bottle perfectly clean and sweet; and to preserve the milk from becoming sour.   You will remember that the young infant is an embryo school-child; good advice to the mother or elder sister may result in sending better material to your school in the future.

Clothing the Child. — The object to be sought by clothing is to keep a uniform layer of air in contact with the body and the limbs.   Dress may be well arranged without necessarily costing more than garments ill adapted to health.   It is preferable to have woollen garments next to the body; but whatever their material, the make is also important; garments should not be tight anywhere at the collar or at the waist; in the winter especially the undergarment should come up to the neck with a low collar band, and the sleeves should be continued below the elbow.   It is hardly necessary to dwell on the fact that constriction of the waist with a view to improve the figure is a foolish imprudence. In wet weather children should if possible change their boots on entering the school.

Though it is not possible to describe here the means of early recognition of all diseases of children of school age, it may be useful to say a few words about some of those more commonly seen in the school which should be early detected by teachers with a view to prevent the spread of infection, and others which may arise or be observed during school attendance.

Ophthalmia. — Is sometimes called "blight in the eyes." The membrane lining the eyelids and covering the white portion of the eye ball may become red and inflamed, producing an unhealthy thick yellow-ish discharge, which is highly infectious. This form of inflammation of the eyes is called ophthalmia, and is one of the greatest causes of blindness. Any child with secretion coming from its eyes, should not use a pocket handkerchief, but the eyes may be cleansed with portions of cotton wool, which should then be burnt at once to destroy the infectious matter. In cleansing the eyes, wet bits of soft rag in warm water then drip the wet on to the eyes, with the lids separated by your thumb and finger, so as to wash away all discharges. The discharge is very contagious; be most careful that no particle finds its way to your own eyes; burn every bit of rag after it has been used, and wash your hands in a infecting fluid.   If the child is kept in school, constant care must be taken to keep the eyes clean ; but the child should be isolated if possible and placed under medical care.

Ulcer on the Front of the Eye (Cornea). — Children with such ulcers cannot face the light, and keep their eyes screwed up : often they get the bad eye tied up with a handkerchief to exclude the light.   This disease mostly occurs in children of poor health and low nutrition.   An ulcer or depressed white spot may be seen in the front of the eye, often at the centre or sight of the eye ; if this does not quickly heal, it will leave a permanent white patch, which will ever after interfere with the sight.

Summer Diarrhœa is very frequent and very fatal among young children in the hot weather.   Such an epidemic occurs in towns almost every year, when the mean temperature of the air rises above $63°$ F.   The general sanitation of the home is the best preventive measure ; the rooms should be kept very clean and well ventilated, urge great cleanliness and daily bathing of children or sponging with cold water.   Children ought not to be allowed to eat either unripe or decomposing fruit ; and at this time of the year, in particular, great care should be taken as to keeping milk sweet ; it should be all scalded before being used.

Chicken-pox begins with slight rise of temperature, and on the second day a small number of reddish pimples appear, some of which soon become watery heads : it spreads rapidly among children.

Measles begin with all the symptoms of a common cold, running of the eyes and nose, hoarseness of voice, and a rise of temperature. The eruption on the skin appears about the third day on the face, neck, and arms. It is extremely infectious and leads to many deaths among children.

Scarlet Fever begins with sore throat and a rise of temperature. The red rash comes out on the body, the arms, and the face on the second day of illness. It is very infectious and dangerous ; when the fever is gone, the skin is left rough, and fine powder peels off from it, which is the source of infection. The child who has recovered from scarlet fever should not be received at school till all peeling of the skin of the hands has ceased ; baths should be used with disinfectants during convalescence. If a case of scarlet fever is found in school, the books and papers the child has touched in the schoolroom should be burnt. The infection is very easily carried from the home where a child is ill to the school by a child not yet ill.

Diphtheria. — The child may complain of sore throat, and the voice be partially lost ; while in bad cases among young children an unpleasant discharge may come down the nose and accumulate on the upper lip ; this discharge is very infectious. The temperature is not high in diphtheria, but the glands under the jaw may enlarge rapidly.

Taking the Temperature. — If a child is flushed or ill, complaining of pains or headaches, and looks like sickening for an illness, it is useful that you should take his temperature with a thermometer. The natural temperature of the body is uniform, and in health stands at $98\frac{1}{2}°$ F. Every school should be provided with a clinical thermometer. Place the bulb, which contains the mercury, in the mouth, under the tongue, with the lips gently closed around the stem, and keep it there three minutes; when you remove it, notice how high the mercury stands in the stem; if it is above 100° F., the child is ill and unfit for the schoolroom.

Some diseases are contagious : the inflammation of ophthalmia and diphtheria produces secretions which if they reach a healthy child may reproduce the same disease in him. The contagious material may be said to convey the germs of the disease. So with other catching diseases, as ringworm of the head. In scarlet fever the dust from the skin of the convalescent patient conveys the disease, so the clothes must be disinfected. In measles, scarlet fever, whooping-cough, the poison may pass through the air from the patient to the healthy children; hence isolation is necessary. Always disinfect your hands after touching any patient with a catching disease.

Simple disinfection may be required in the schoolroom, as for your hands after you have touched the face of a child with ophthalmia or one believed to have a fever. For this purpose a few drops of Condy's fluid (permanganate of potash) just to colour the water in a hand-basin, or a solution of carbolic acid 1 in 40 parts, may be used; a weak solution of corrosive sublimate (1–3000) may be used to wash over the floor after infection.

Chorea, or St. Vitus's dance, is frequent during school age, and is more common among girls than boys. This occurs in some of the bright, well-made children; it is characterised by weakness and a number of awkward twitches and movements, while the girl becomes somewhat childish in manner. The onset is usually gradual, the girl becomes clumsy, things drop from her hands, as the fingers open spontaneously, the hand when held out assume the nervous posture, while the fingers twitch, there may be facial grimaces, usually about the mouth, and the eyes are much moved; the shoulders may often be drawn up and down, and other abnormal nerve-signs are observable. Though many spontaneous movements thus occur, they are at first partially under control, and momentary quietness may be produced by arresting the child's attention. These children have often suffered from rheumatism or pains in joints and limbs, with some swelling of one knee after fatigue or what are vaguely called "growing pains". Another important point is that these children are almost always below their normal weight, often losing a pound in weight or more in a week.

Case 50. A girl thirteen years of age; in Standard VI.; after a slight attack of sore throat, became very irritable; she was unable to write properly or hold her book straight and began to drop things from her hands. She left school, but was not laid up. When seen at the hospital, her weight was much below the normal; when she held out her hands, there was much movement seen at the elbows and wrists, while the fingers twitched; imitation of movements was fairly performed, but with many extra-movements, not controlled through her eyes. At the end of a month's treatment she had gained four pounds in weight, and the movements subsided; she made a good recovery. There was disease of the heart, as so often is present in these cases, and that remained.

Epilepsy is a grave disease; you may occasionally see an epileptic attack, but more often you will be told that a child, who otherwise should be at school, has had a fit. An epileptic fit is a sudden seizure; a momentary pallor of the face is succeeded by loss of consciousness, the patient falls, the hands are clenched; the face is distorted and becomes blue or black with congestion, while the convulsion spreads to the limbs. After such an attack the child is drowsy and needs rest. In some cases the attacks are much less severe, only momentary unconsciousness occurring without convulsion (*petit mal*). It is difficult to say what should be done for such children; they need training with education, and do best when fully occupied in the country; to leave them untrained doing nothing through childhood is very unwise.

Rickets is so frequently seen among children who live in towns that the indications of this condition ought to be known to you; the signs you will see are mostly in the bones, the head, and in growth. These cases are common in the infant school, and more boys than girls are affected. They are short for their age and remain stunted, the head is often large and ill shapen, the forehead bulging or projecting on either side; the legs may be bowed and knock-kneed, making the child a bad walker. In a young child, say three or four years, the ends of the bones of the arms just above the wrists are usually large. The chest is " pigeon-breasted," thrust forward in the middle line, and pressed in at the sides. Rickets is largely due to feeding babies with bread and other farinaceous food in place of milk; these children are delicate, they grow up stunted, and about one-third of them prove to be dull pupils; rickets could probably be prevented in any child by attention to the rules of health.

A well-arranged schoolhouse and classrooms will do much towards the culture of physical and mental health. Good lighting gives cheerfulness and is better for sight and for teaching; when possible it is better that the desks be arranged so that with a unilateral light, the windows are on the left hand of the children; the windows should be kept bright and the blinds drawn well up; if windows are on two sides of the room, curtains may be wanted to regulate the light.

The children should in wet weather change their boots on entering school: the cloak-room should be arranged with a space for each child to prevent the mixing of the clothes. Lavatories are often badly constructed; for a large school it is safer to have no wash-basins, a stream of water from a tap to wash in tends to prevent contagion, and the use of the lavatory should be supervised. It is much to be desired that school children should be encouraged to use the public swimming baths, now so frequently provided in towns.

In considering the health of the children I would refer you to what has been said in former chapters as to sight; and as to defective hearing in the mouth-breathers. Remember that children, small in growth, small-headed, or with any defect in development of the body, are apt to become delicate and dull mentally, so that the views of the parents of the dull pupil who object to long home lessons for the child may be reasonable; this will lead you to study the child as to both his mental and physical status. Other points concerning mental and physical health are put forward in the Propositions on Childhood (Chapter XIII.).

The care of health in delicate children does not necessarily imply giving up their training; there are many young children, delicate for a time without

disease, besides those described as " nervous children."
I think it would be of service to the teacher, if some
account of the child's condition and physical and
brain defects were prepared by a medical man, showing
in what points that child may require special care. In
the case of all delicate children the teacher's own
examination should be some guide, as is explained in
Chapter XI., and the points given for the observation of
children will aid in health culture.

When visiting a school in East London with one
of the managers, and glancing over the children as
they stood or worked in their classes, several cases
of illness and disease were soon apparent. Two or
three had obvious defects of vision, capable of easy
correction by glasses, and one had disease of his eyes,
which threatened to destroy his sight completely before manhood. This was pointed out to the head-
master and a ticket for the neighbouring hospital
was offered.

School hygiene in its mental aspects and the culture of brain-healthiness among children generally, as
well as in certain groups subnormal, is a subject
dealt with throughout this work, and includes the
cultivation of good brain-power and the avoidance of
an amount of fatigue leading to exhaustion

It can hardly be said that at present there exists
any established science of mental hygiene ; yet some
good materials are at hand for further developments

of exact mental science and the study of child-mind. It seems to me essential to a scientific mental hygiene of childhood, that we should be better acquainted with its types and varieties. Some of these have been described, but it must be remembered that the classes I have described are mostly children subnormal in some point, amounting to 20 per cent of the school children seen by me. We want a mental hygiene for childhood at large, and subsections dealing with certain groups. There may be mental and motor fatigue; the general signs of fatigue which you may observe have here been described. Much stress has been laid on the avoidance of fatigue, or at any rate such continued fatigue as amounts to exhaustion. The laws of mental fatigue are not the same as those of muscular fatigue. The nerve-system is in part an apparatus for the storage and distribution of energy; it is further an apparatus consisting of a great number of parts or brain-centres, which are separately under control of the senses; their coördination and coacting represent the physical basis of mental processes.

The subject of mental fatigue has been investigated by Dr. Leo Burgerstein of Vienna, Dr. Rivers of Cambridge University, and others. Dr. Burgerstein observed with care and accuracy the effects of one hour's mental occupation, as indicated by the mental mistakes made. The principal tests used were in addition and multiplication of figures. He came to the conclusion that the working power rises and falls during the time of an ordinary lesson, and that it is not well to let lessons last longer than three-quarters of an hour; advising to interrupt the continuation of lessons by pauses of about a quarter of an hour, so as to have the children's brain rested, the body moved, and the school-room air changed.

CHAPTER XIII

PROPOSITIONS CONCERNING CHILDHOOD

Proposition I. — *The main classes of defect among school children include a larger proportion of boys than girls.*

Evidence as to the truth of this statement is sufficiently afforded in Table VII., which shows that a larger proportion of boys than girls present defect in development, abnormal nerve-signs, and mental dulness ; but the girls present the largest proportion of delicate cases ; this is in accordance with common experience during school-life. Still it has been shown that it is only the girls with development defect that are so prone to be delicate, not all girls.

Again : although it is here stated that the proportion of girls in any way below the normal as indicated by any main class of defect, except delicacy, is smaller than among boys ; still, when a girl has some defect, it is often of more real importance than a similar condition in a boy. See Proposition VI.

The general rule, that defectiveness falls mostly on the male sex, holds good also in adult life, as seen among the classes with physical infirmities, the blind, deaf, and mentally deranged from childhood; so also for criminals and paupers according to the English Census and other official returns.

I have shown elsewhere (see "Statistical Journal," March, 1896, London), that a larger proportion of girls than boys present two or more classes of defect associated in the same case; and their condition is worse than that of children with one class of defect only. A child with an ill-shapen head or palate may have no other defect; but if, in addition, he become delicate, he is at a disadvantage. So a boy only dull, while strong and active, may get his living; but if he is also slow in action and of poor health, he is likely to become dependent

Proposition II. — *The main classes of defect among school children are much associated in the groups of cases; such associations vary with sex, age, and environment.*

Evidence as to this proposition is given in Table VIII. Developmental defects are much associated in children with abnormal nerve-signs, low nutrition, and mental dulness. A child presenting a developmental defect only, e.g. a narrow palate, defect of external ears or other features, may be at no personal disadvantage; it is in conditions commonly associated therewith that harm arises.

So each class of defect if unaccompanied by any other deficiency may not give rise to any serious trouble; but when defects are associated in the same case, they produce harm in life.

Taking all classes of defect together, the association of two or more classes of defect in the same case is less commonly found in school children at eleven years and over, than at seven years and under: this fact seems to indicate a favourable evolution of childhood during school life.

It is the children with developmental defects that acquire the most association with other classes of defect as time goes on, developing abnormal nerve-signs, mental dulness, and low nutrition; they have a low power of resistance to an adverse environment. Probably their heredity is a part of the causation of this condition; but much may be done during school-life to prevent evils arising.

In this class of children there appears to be disproportioning in bodily development, and associated therewith delicacy of body, and proneness to disorderly brain-action. As a group, in an institution, such children acquire more abnormal signs than in the day school, but grow fatter.

It is shown in Proposition VII. that good physical training has some effect in lessening the proportion of children acquiring associated defects.

Co-relation. — It is in the co-relations of defects that new information is mostly to be looked for, supplying evidence as to the real significance of the defects respectively, and as to their causation. Inasmuch as it has been shown by the comparison of groups of schools that the co-relation of the main classes of defects varies as to degree with the character of the environment, it is advisable to determine the percentage of co-relations of defects upon similar groups of cases under different environment.[1] To some extent this has been done by giving the co-relations of the main classes of defects and individual defects, as seen in children in day schools and in residential schools. The difference in the numerical values of these co-relations, under different environments are, in some degree, a measure of their effect

Proposition III. — *Children with developmental defects often present also abnormal nerve-signs, and are delicate and dull.*

Not only are these developmental cases frequently pale, thin, and delicate in school-life; as infants they are very delicate, while from being more common among boys than girls they add largely to the male infant mortality in the first year; the cases that survive form a large proportion of the delicate, dull, and nervous children in schools, especially among girls

Of the children with developmental defects :

The proportion of these with abnormal nerve-signs associated rises in the age-groups up to ten years, being higher among boys; the proportion continues t

[1] See published Report on Childhood.

R

rise slightly for girls, but falls with the boys at eleven years and over.

The proportion of those who are pale, thin, delicate, is highest at seven years and under, being twelve per cent higher among girls than boys; this proportion falls greatly to eleven years, but at all ages remains higher with girls.

Proposition IV. — *Children with indications of brain-disorderliness*, i.e. *abnormal nerve-signs, are often dull pupils.*

The proportion of children with abnormal nerve-signs who are dull varies but little with age and sex. Among all children abnormal nerve-signs are intimately associated with mental dulness.

These children are seen from various points of view. Teachers see the pupil's awkward habits, listlessness, slouching gait, slow action and response, irregularities in movements of the hands, wandering eyes, or other "abnormal nerve-signs."

Take 100 boys and 100 girls with such nerve-signs : on the basis of the average obtained — 18 of the boys are probably pale, thin, delicate ; and 40 dull at lessons : among the girls 29 are delicate and 42 dull. The status of these girls is worse than that of the boys, and they show more general delicacy. It is well to adopt a method of physical training, adapted to remove abnormal nerve-signs and their attendant troubles.

The doctor in charge of the child may well bear in mind that though a period of treatment is necessary for the removal of a brain weakness or disorder, at the same time care should be taken if possible that the child is so managed and employed or trained, as to prevent any unnecessary amount of mental deteriora tion. Cases of chorea, paralysis, epilepsy, if left with out any appropriate training, tend to grow up dull and mentally feeble.

In the fact of the frequent association of abnormal nerve-signs and mental dulness evidence is afforded that such points of ill-balance and defective action are really indications of brain-disorderliness and want of proper action. When good training removes such signs, the brain is brighter for mental action Here we see a method of combating mental dulness

In dealing with a child exceptionally dull, one of the first practical points is to indicate to the teacher the nerve-signs present and the means of removing them by appropriate management and training. This is a reason why teachers should learn to observe and describe chil dren, that they may know what to do for them

Proposition V. — *Dull pupils are often d.. te   indications of brain-disorderliness, i.e. abnormal ner. signs.*

Dull and backward pupils are often pale, thin, deli cate. This condition of low nutrition app ... t ...

in part, a cause of mental dulness, and acts more powerfully with girls than with boys at all ages ; such low nutrition among dull pupils is seen mostly in those seven years and under, being three times as frequent among dull children at that age, as at eleven years and over.

Although it is thus shown that a state of low nutrition is probably a cause of mental dulness, it appears that the brain-disorderliness indicated by abnormal nerve-signs is much more commonly a cause of dulness. Abnormal nerve-signs are more frequently seen among dull boys than dull girls at all ages ; they are less frequent among the children seven years and under than above that age.

These facts should be appreciated both by teachers and parents. The teacher naturally notes the dull pupils. If we take 100 dull boys and 100 dull girls of all ages according to the estimate made: of the boys 15 are probably delicate, and of the girls 19. The difficulties and requirements of dull boys and dull girls differ. Again: of the boys, 57 probably present abnormal nerve-signs, and 52 of the girls. Many of the dull children do not move their eyes in looking at objects, their response in action is slow and inexact, as well as in speech : they are lacking in spontaneity, ill-balanced in limbs and body, listless and slouching.

Physical training, adapted to remove in detail each

abnormal nerve-sign, may do much to remove their inert and disorderly brain-action and render them brighter mentally. It is clear from the facts given that dull pupils if accumulated in a class need more than an increased amount of instruction; they are many of them delicate children, needing brain-training as well as purely mental culture.

Proposition VI. — *Girls with developmental defect or brain-disorderliness are more apt to receive harm and less good from their environment than boys.*

Contrasting boys and girls, it may be pointed out that there are certain differences which may be classed as :

(1) Developmental.

(2) Brain-conditions : including mental dulness and incoördinated action.

(3) Effects of the environment and interaction of effects.

(*a*) Physical, (*b*) Mental and moral.

(4) Effects of disease.

Cases with developmental defect are more frequent in males, but under the effects of their environment the girls tend to acquire nerve-disorder, mental dulness, and low nutrition in larger proportion than the boys. See Propositions I. and II.

Imbeciles are more frequent among boys, but the mortality is higher with imbecile girls

In school the proportion of those who are dull at eleven years and older is higher with girls. It should, however, be pointed out that the regularity of school attendance of girls appears to be always lower than with boys.

These cases though less frequent among girls may lead to very serious results, and if not duly cared for, they may be permanently injured in mental and physical power by inappropriate education and management or by neglect.

Cases with Brain-disorderliness indicated by Abnormal Nerve-signs. — These cases are more frequent among boys, but the proportion of those who are mentally dull is slightly higher among girls, and 16 per cent of these girls are also pale, thin, delicate, as against 12 per cent of the boys. The outcome is that these girls are more likely to fall into permanent ill-health than the boys; thus more boys than girls in school present finger-twitching, but more girls acquire chorea and anæmia.

Analogous facts may be quoted: insanity may be slightly more frequent among males — the rate of discharge from asylums (by death or recovery) is higher among males, the proportion of chronic cases is higher among females. Criminals of the male sex are far more frequent than females, but "criminals convicted 10 times and over" are twice as frequent among females. Among criminal lunatics, murder, as apart from infanticide, is much more common among females. Dull boys are more frequent than dull girls in school; but the number of illiterate brides still exceeds the number of illiterate bridegrooms, though the disproportion is happily decreasing by the advance of women.

It appears that female brains, when "disorderly," whether mentally dull, lunatic, or criminal, are more apt to remain disorderly than male brains. This shows the importance of preventing such disorderliness in school-life; and I would again draw attention to the probable evils that result from the irregular school attendance of girls.

Males and females do not present with similar frequency:

(1) Constitutional or congenital defects

(2) Diseases and acquired pathological conditions

(3) Their reaction under ill effects of environment differ.

(4) The effects of environment, suitable to one sex, are not always equally suitable to the other

It appears that constitutional congenital defect, while more common in males, reacts less unfavourably under the environment in them, than among females; in the latter, the environment often causes additional evils, while among the population at large we see more early death among males, and the woman's expectancy of life exceeds that of the man.

Proposition VII. — *The effects of good physical training in school are to diminish the number of cases with signs of brain-disorderliness and the number of dull children.*

Evidence is available from comparison of reports on children seen in schools, where good physical training was provided, in contrast with a large school, where no such training was given. In the school without physical training the proportion of both boys and girls with abnormal nerve-signs was higher, and a larger proportion of the boys were reported by the teachers as dull pupils. This cannot be attributed to the Developmental cases or to Low Nutrition, as their proportion was lower than in the other schools; it must, I think, be ascribed to the absence of physical training. Again, in this school the children who had some developmental defects showed a higher association with both abnormal nerve-signs and mental dulness, than those under a system of good physical training.

It may be inferred that physical training tends to improve the brain-condition of children, preventing or removing disorderliness in motor and in mental action, and promotes healthy activity in both directions; this applies not only to children perfectly well made in body but also to those in some slight degree below normal.

TABLE VII

Based on 50,000 children seen in day schools, mostly in or near London (1892–94): viz.: 26,287 boys, 23,713 girls. Showing the total number of children with each main class of defect and groups of defect, and the percentages on the number of children seen at all ages. The last column gives the number of girls per 100 boys per combined group.

MAIN CLASSES OF DEFECT AND GROUPS OF DEFECT	NUMBER IN GROUPS		PERCENTAGE ON NUMBER OF CHILDREN SEEN		NUMBER OF GIRLS PER 100 BOYS PER COMBINED GROUP	
	Boys	Girls	Boys	Girls	On total examined	On total with a defect
A All children with developmental defect	2108	1618	8.8	6.8	78	95
B All children with abnormal nerve signs	2852	2015	10.8	8.5	78	96
C All children with low nutrition	749	779	2.8	3.2	114	140
D All children mentally ...	2074	1614	7.9	6.9	87	107
AB ...	887	587	3.4	2.5	73	90
...	374	428	1.4	1.8	127	150
...	853	727	3.3	3.1	91	111
...	351	315	1.1	1.4	10	129
...	115	804	4.5	3.6	8.	98
...	351	313	1.3	1.3	115	131
...	143	150			1.	142
...	41		1.2		1.	102
...	171	182	0.6		122	150
...	155	141			28	13
...	8.	72	1	0.1	12	130
...	25	331	1.2	1	132	130

TABLE VIII

Based on 50,000 children seen in day schools, mostly in or near London (1892–94); viz.: 26,287 boys, 23,713 girls. Showing the co-relation or association of the main classes of defect observed in children.

The table is arranged in four columns, giving the percentages for children in the age-groups and at all ages. The percentages are taken on the number with the main class of defect.

Thus: Of all cases with development defect at all ages, 38.4 per cent of the boys and 49.9 per cent of the girls were mentally dull.

Of all the dull children at all ages, 57.6 per cent of the boys and 52.6 per cent of the girls also presented abnormal nerve-signs.

	7 Years and under		Age 8–10		Age 11 and over		All Ages		
	Boys	Girls	Boys	Girls	Boys	Girls	Boys	Girls	
A									All cases with developmental defect. Boys, 2308; girls, 1618
AB	31.7	28.5	43.3	41.4	40.5	44.0	38.4	36.2	Per cent with abnormal nerve-signs
AC	22.7	35.0	16.0	22.1	7.5	15.0	16.2	26.3	Per cent with low nutrition
AD	36.6	40.8	41.2	46.6	37.1	51.1	38.4	44.9	Per cent with mental dulness
B									All cases with abnormal nerve-signs. Boys, 2853; girls, 2015
AB	35.1	41.2	30.6	28.0	28.3	21.4	31.0	29.1	Per cent with developmental defect
BC	19.6	27.4	11.3	15.2	7.5	10.2	12.3	16.6	Per cent with low nutrition
BD	43.3	47.0	42.6	41.9	39.6	40.4	41.8	42.6	Per cent with mental dulness
C									All cases with low nutrition. Boys, 749; girls, 770
AC	52.5	66.1	51.0	50.4	39.3	35.5	49.9	55.5	Per cent with developmental defect
BC	41.1	36.0	51.1	51.1	56.4	49.9	47.1	43.5	Per cent with abnormal nerve-signs
CD	43.6	42.0	44.8	40.7	37.6	35.6	43.1	40.5	Per cent with mental dulness
D									All dull children. Boys, 2077; girls, 1635
AD	45.9	55.1	43.3	42.6	38.6	34.9	42.8	44.4	Per cent with developmental defect
BD	49.0	44.1	63.4	56.6	59.1	56.7	57.6	52.6	Per cent with abnormal nerve-signs
CD	23.6	30.1	14.8	16.3	7.5	10.2	15.5	19.0	Per cent with low nutrition

INDEX

251

S

www.ingramcontent.com/pod-product-compliance
Lightning Source LLC
Chambersburg PA
CBHW030339270326
41926CB00009B/888